D0093298

CLOSE TO THE BONE

Life-Threatening Illness and the Search for Meaning

JEAN SHINODA BOLEN, M.D.

SCRIBNER

SCRIBNER
1230 Avenue of the Americas
New York, NY 10020

Designed by Margery Cantor
Set in Adobe Garamond and Poetica

Manufactured in the United States of America
1   3   5   7   9   10   8   6   4   2

Library of Congress Cataloging-in-Publication Data
Bolen, Jean Shinoda.
Close to the bone : life-threatening illness and the search for meaning /
Jean Shinoda Bolen.
p. cm.
Includes index.
1. Sick—Psychology.   I. Title.
R726.5.B65   1996
616'.001'9—dc20   96-26236
CIP
ISBN 0-684-82237-7

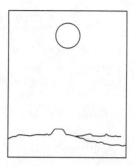

CONTENTS

Introduction   9

1   Close to the Bone: Illness and the Soul   13

2   The Ground Gives Way Under Us   23

3   Harbinger of Truth   40

4   Like Green Meat on a Hook   53

5   Procrustean Dismemberment   63

6   Illness as a Turning Point   76

7   Sometimes We Need a Story   91

8   Soul Connections   110

9   Summoning Angels: Prayer   129

10   Prescribing Imagination   143

Contents

11   Rituals: Enacting Myth   157

12   Helping Each Other   179

13   Musings   195

Acknowledgments   211

Sources   213

Index   215

Close to the Bone

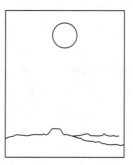

INTRODUCTION

The Chinese pictograph for *crisis* is comprised of the ideograms for "danger" and "opportunity." Every life-threatening illness is a major crisis for everyone concerned that shakes the foundations of previous assumptions. Such a crisis is not restricted to the person with the illness, nor is it just about the fate of a body. A life-threatening condition throws all aspects of life for the patient and all significant relationships into a time of turmoil and transition. Life-threatening illness is a crisis for the soul. When death and disability come close, it is indeed a time of danger and opportunity, which raises questions about the meaning of life and tests the bonds of relationships.

This book grew out of a series of lectures and workshops about illness as a descent of the soul into the underworld and the healing that can result. The central message that illness is a soul experience was one of the inspirations for a series of conferences for women surviving cancer, called "Healing Journeys: Cancer as a Turning Point," along with Lawrence LeShan's ground-breaking book, whose title inspired the sec-

ond part of the conference name. Cancer as a turning point was the
perspective of the four organizers, three of whom had been diagnosed
and treated for cancer of the breast.

I have accompanied family members, friends, and patients through
illnesses and hospitalizations that were descents into the underworld.
The terrain is very familiar, though the gateway of physical illness is not
as familiar as the psychological entry points that bring people on a soul
path into a Jungian analysis with me.

Whether the life-threatening illness is psychological or physical,
when depression colors or influences thought and action, people often
give up on themselves and on the future. It is then not enough to treat
a depression only with medications, or only pay attention to the physical signs and symptoms of disease, when giving up on life having any
meaning, now or in the future, is the underlying life-or-death issue.

The parallels between psychiatric and physical life-threatening illnesses are easy for me to see because I have straddled both worlds.
Before I was a psychiatrist and even now as an analyst, I am, in some
essential way, still a physician. Medical school and a rotating internship
in a large county hospital were an initiation, not just an education. To
be a doctor of the body or of the psyche is to be at those border cross-
ings between ordinary life and life thereafter. A life-threatening illness
brings an end to a phase of life, as it may to life itself. The doctor of the
body or of the psyche is a witness to and a participant in the outcome.

A life-threatening illness has the impact of a stone hitting the still
surface of a lake, sending concentric rings of disturbance out, as feelings, thoughts, and reactions radiate out from this center. It impacts
relationships, it stirs the depths of others, it potentially brings the
patient and those who are affected "close to the bone," into the prox-
imity of the soul. Soul questions arise about the meaning of life when
the mind is ill or the body is ailing. Healing and recovery may depend
as much or more upon a deepening of relationships and connection to
one's own soul and spiritual life, as on medical or psychiatric expertise.

I have learned over and over again that a life-threatening illness is soul-shaking for everyone involved, that it provides us an opportunity to get intimations and intuitions about why we are here, and what and who really matters. It is this experience, and the archetypal underpinning provided by mythology, that is the soul of the book

I hope this book will be an inner companion during a time of descent or difficulty. Maybe it will come to you through synchronicity to affirm what you intuitively know, and to support you to do whatever it is that will heal you. I can imagine it being read aloud, a portion or a chapter. I hope that it opens the way for significant conversations with others, and to rich internal dialogues with yourself.

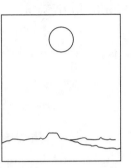

CLOSE TO THE BONE:
ILLNESS AND THE SOUL

I n noisy wards and crowded waiting rooms of county hospitals and clinics, in quiet private rooms in medical center pavilions or in well-appointed waiting rooms, examining rooms, or offices, wherever there are patients, there are long moments of silence, pauses, sometimes preceded by a sigh, a transient stillness when the air feels heavier. When the eyes of the patient or others who are there turn inward. When someone retreats inside as others chatter, or seems to be somewhere else even as the doctor is explaining something important. Sometimes I have glimpsed that same look with its attendant quiet on the face of a doctor or nurse. Occasionally, a room suddenly, collectively, goes silent in this same deep way; when this happened, the ancient Greeks would observe: "Hermes has entered." Hermes was the messenger god and the guide of souls to the underworld; dreams and divination came under his auspices. Today, when that hush happens, someone is apt to break the silence with "An angel has come." A subtle perceptible shift in the air unaccountably occurs that people from ancient times to the present have attributed to the presence of invisible winged messengers from the eternal world. In these moments, the persona or face we wear for the ordinary world to see drops away and the mind is empty of its preoccupations and responsibilities, and we are with soul.

Illness and the Soul

The reality and possibility of serious illness evokes soul from the first moment it registers: it might be after hearing a report that something serious was found on the X-ray or more sophisticated scans or in the specimen sent to the lab, or after an illness announced itself with the sudden onset of acute pain, loss of consciousness, or bleeding, or after the discovery of a suspicious lump or discolored area, or after surviving a suicide attempt or a disabling injury. Whenever or however that line from health to illness is crossed, we enter this realm of soul. Illness is both soul-shaking and soul-evoking for the patient and for all others for whom the patient matters. We lose an innocence, we know vulnerability, we are no longer who we were before this event, and we will never be the same. We are in uncharted terrain, and there is no turning back. Illness is a profound soul event, and yet this is virtually ignored and unaddressed. Instead, everything seems to be focused on the part of the body that is sick, damaged, failing, or out of control.

A hospital has much in common with an auto body repair shop. It is there with its staff of specialists to diagnose, fix, or replace what it can of the physical body to get it running again. The patient and those accompanying the patient through this crisis are considered to behave well if they do not get in the way of whatever the doctors want to do with the ailing body. Troublesome patients (or their troublesome significant others) ask questions, want to understand what is wrong and why a particular treatment and not something else has been selected, bother doctors with requests, or don't respond properly. The medical setting is one in which there is a definite line of authority, with the doctor in charge and others responsible for carrying out orders. A good patient like a good soldier is one who cooperates or obeys orders. Especially when cancer is the diagnosis but in many other conditions as well, the doctor's perspective is often similar to a general at war: the disease is the enemy to be fought, with the body of the patient the battleground.

Threshold Between Life and Death

When something is wrong with our bodies, we want whatever is wrong to be fixed. When something destructive is going on in our bodies, we want the disease to be stopped. We go to doctors and to hospitals with the expectation that they will take care of our bodies. That the soul might also be engaged is not our expectation. Yet, a life-threatening illness calls to the soul, taps into spiritual resources, and can be an initiation into the soul realm for the patient and for anyone else who is touched by the mystery that accompanies the possibility of death. When life is lived at the edge—in the border realm between life and death—it is a *liminal* time and place. *Liminal* comes from the Latin word for "threshold." It is not an everyday word; it is one whose meaning I want to evoke out of the remembered experience of the reader and the collective memory of the human race, which we all have access to. Whenever we participate in something that will change us, and change how others relate to us—as when we marry, are inducted into the armed forces or ordained, become a doctor, or survive an ordeal—that experience is a liminal one. Whenever we are initiated into knowing something we did not know before on a body level—for example, through sexual intercourse or pregnancy—we cross a threshold. Here the mystical, spiritual, or psychic awareness of what is happening, however, determines its significance as a soul experience. So it is with a life-threatening illness, which similarly happens in and to the body and yet can profoundly affect the soul.

Illness, especially when death is a possibility, makes us acutely aware of how precious life is and how precious a particular life is. Priorities shift. We may see the truth of what matters, who matters, and what we have been doing with our lives and have to decide what to do—now that we know. Significant relationships are tested and either come through strengthened or fail. Pain and fear bring us to our knees in prayer. Our spiritual and religious convictions or the lack of them are called into question. Illness is an ordeal for both body and soul, and a time when healing of either or both can result.

Once upon a time, or so it seemed, potentially fatal illnesses were unexpected tragic events that happened to young children and terminal illnesses were mostly chronic conditions that afflicted the elderly. Diagnostic tests and biopsies have made it possible to diagnose life-threatening illnesses earlier and treat them aggressively; so much so that invasive treatments can be health and life endangering themselves. Midlife now presents the possibility of death and disability for far too many people. AIDS and cancer are claiming so many in their prime adult years that many of us feel that midlife is a medical battlefield with people dropping around us; for those of us in the health professions the impact of numbers is even greater. Life-threatening illnesses are striking close to home. One may be threatening your spouse, your lover, your son or your daughter, your parent, your friend, or you.

To be a passive, obedient patient or the terrain on which a battle is fought by the medical profession goes against the grain of people who question authority, see value in alternative viewpoints, and understand that body and psyche are related. Whether as patient or as a person with love and responsibility for the patient, there are life-and-death consequences to the choices we make or allow others to make. To act out of fear or out of trust, to go with intuition or against it, to do what we know is right for us when it upsets someone else—issues that are life issues are made all the more crucial when death or recovery may depend upon what we decide. Moreover, if the battle for a medical cure is lost, doctors often abandon the field, all but avoiding the patient, who is now a reminder of defeat.

Illness as a Psychological Ordeal

The travails of being a patient and the physical illness together are an ordeal that can have a transformative effect on the soul. Psychological stress is a major part of the ordeal through which the soul must pass. When the possibility of a serious illness unexpectedly arises on a routine examination, or there is an onset of symptoms, or there is a need to be hospitalized, we may be assailed by fears and vulnerabilities. We fear—with or without justification—that we may never be our former healthy selves, ever again. Those close to the patient may also be having these or similar concerns, or be having them when the patient is not. Thoughts are shaped by how we perceive what is happening to us or to someone near and dear, every bit as much and sometimes even more so, than by objective information. Depending upon our psychological makeup, under such circumstances we tend to live in the present or in the future as we foresee it. If a serious illness is a potential that will only be known after the biopsy or after the workup, a person who lives in the present can often put dire possibilities easily out of mind: an attitude of "why borrow trouble?" comes naturally. A future-oriented person, on the other hand, especially one who worries or is aware of the likelihood and magnitude of the situation, may have the patient practically dead and buried before the results are in. Stress may be virtually absent for one, and off the chart for the other. When someone is in the throes of pain, limitations, weakness, or nausea, the awfulness of the moment may not only be all there is, but all there ever will be for that person, while another person faced with the same symptoms may experience this as part of a difficult time that will pass. When pain is not relieved, or obsessive negative thoughts crowd the mind, they leave little room to attend to the concerns of the soul.

Soul Moments

For soul to be heard, the mind must be still. Then thoughts and feelings can arise as if from a deep well within us. Often these thoughts and feelings are not shared. When they are, the soul looks outward for a moment, and we hope that we can truly share the depth into which illness is taking us. We wonder if we should die, will our lives have been worthwhile? What do we regret doing or not having done? What do we still want time for? Do we matter? Do the people in our lives really matter to us? Is there a God? An afterlife? What unfinished business gnaws at us? What long-buried thoughts and memories are coming back to us now? What are our dreams saying?

When we voice concerns and content such as these, we are baring our soul. At such moments, we are as if naked, and all too often when we speak of such matters, the impulse of others is to hurriedly cover up our words with a thin layer of reassurance—to which we respond by withdrawing. Revealing matters of the soul makes those who dwell in shallower waters uncomfortable. Soul-searching questions are those that people who are addicted to work or to alcohol or to superficial activities are warding off by their addictions. They do not want to be exposed to their own deep questions, as voiced by us.

Sometimes, we are caught looking inward, feeling something move in our own depths—a thought, a memory, emotion, an intuition, wisdom—and someone says, "A penny for your thoughts?" And we retreat self-consciously. Or this time we speak our concerns aloud, and there is joy at finding a soul friend. A soul-level friend is a sanctuary, a person to whom we can tell the truth of what we feel or know or perceive. When something is expressed at a soul level, it is not something for the other to fix or minimize or deny or take personally; what is said and felt needs to be received, heard, accepted, held—as in a womb space, where the insights into ourselves and what matters to us can incubate, grow, and develop fully into consciousness.

Those moments of stillness when the eyes seem to turn inward are pregnant silences, times when we are communing with our deeper thoughts or perceptions or holding a feeling or an image that can be all too fleeting; the mood shifts, and holding on to what for a moment we had a grasp on, can be gone like a dream fragment.

The premise of this book is that illness *can be* soul evoking and that the soul realm is one akin to dream or reverie, a source of personal meaning and wisdom that can transform life and heal us. This is not to say that illness is ever welcomed. It can only be retrospectively appreciated by those for whom it was a soul experience, but having a perspective such as this makes the potential of it being so more likely.

Recovery of soul and recovery of the health of the body may occur together or not; healing may occur, and the body may not survive. Life is a terminal condition, after all. It is a matter of when and how we die, not whether we will. Illness takes us out of our ordinary lives and concerns, and confronts us with big questions and the opportunity of tapping into soul knowledge that can transform us and the situation. Prayers that are said and rituals that are done help by focusing us and by tapping into spiritual energies.

At a soul level, we can see clearly what matters and recognize the truth of our personal situation. We know that we are spiritual beings on a human path rather than human beings who may be on a spiritual path. At the soul level we recognize what is sacred and eternal. At the soul level, an illness, even a terminal one, is a potential beginning, a liminal time when we are between the ordinary world and the invisible one.

Soul Questions

I believe that in any particular illness as in every individual life, the soul questions are the same: *What did we come to do? What did we come to learn? What did we come to heal? What and who did we come to love? What are we here for?* Questions to do with the essence of who we are. I believe that illness can be a call to consciousness, a wake-up call some would say, that illness involves a descent into the depths and an exposure to what we fear. I have seen how illness can unearth love and reveal strength of character, and I know that it is truly an opportunity for soul growth. Or not. I believe that stories and myths, dreams and mystical experiences can become more vivid during illnesses, and that integrating soul knowledge from these sources into ordinary life makes life as well as death meaningful.

Close to the Bone

The first time I knew that illness was both a soul and body experience was when I was in my late twenties. I had just begun my psychiatric residency, and took a six-month leave to be with my parents when my father came home to die. My father had lost a long, heroic struggle to overcome the cancer that had defeated his body, and even after medicine could offer no further even ameliorating procedures, his will to live kept him going for many more months. Yet as he died, I saw his eyes open wide, and his face light up with joy. I am convinced that he saw something I could not see, and I trust my perception and deeply appreciate the gift of seeing this. One moment, he was there, the next instant he was gone. Only an empty body remained; his soul had left. His body was warm, and some cells were probably still functioning seconds later, but *he*—his soul—wasn't there anymore. His suffering was over, and the body he left behind was like discarded clothes that were worn and threadbare, familiar and of no further use to the person who once wore them. His face told me that there was something beautiful to look forward to at death, and the period beforehand, in which he took a long time to die, left me with the belief that this period too was important. With an airway, talking was difficult, and in his last months, the inner world seemed to absorb him. Quite possibly, he died after staying as long as he needed to remain, to do whatever it was he had to do at the threshold between this world and the next. Dying people spend their days like newborns do, sleeping and dreaming, and having their basic needs taken care of by others; the dreaming, the reverie, and the moments of clarity and conversation may not only ease the transition but be soul-healing time.

In the intervening years since then, my son, my mother, and closest friends have gone through medical or surgical crises. I found that when a child is going through major surgery, a mother feels the child's and her own vulnerability, perhaps like no other relationship; it also was for a son on the edge of adulthood, an ordeal that had the elements of an initiation into manhood and clearly was a soul journey. The perspective I gave him may have made a difference in how he experienced what he went through. When my eighty-five-year-old mother became too ill to go on, it seemed like the beginning of the end, which is what she and I thought until she made a full recovery and returned to her independent personal and professional life. I think that what I did and said tilted the scales and made a difference, though it was she—at a soul level—who made a decision to live, and her body was able to recover. The medical and surgical crises that my closest friends have gone through affected me in a way that only contemporaries we love can; they bring home to us knowledge of how fleeting our own lives might be.

Everyone who comes to me for analysis or consultation brings me their close-to-the-bone concerns. Drawing on the depth and breadth of this experience convinces me that it is impossible in a lifetime not to be directly or indirectly affected by potentially disabling or potentially fatal illnesses: they can or will happen to us and to others around us. Whether we are the patient or a witness, when illness enters our circle of people, it touches us deeply. Life-threatening illness takes the patients, those who love them, and those who treat them into the realm of soul.

Such illnesses often take us by surprise. The shift between being healthy and being sick can happen to someone so precipitously that it leaves us stunned and without words for the depth into which we are plunged. Words from someone familiar with the territory may provide an orientation; images and metaphors that reflect what I know may be a starting point for inner reflection or the basis of a dialogue on a soul level with someone else. Whether suddenly or gradually, a life-threatening illness has the power to cut through illusions and bring us close to the bone, maybe for the first time in our lives.

To be brought "close to the bone" through the adversity of illness, the closeness of death, and the knowledge that we are not in control of the situation, is to come close to the essence of who we are, both as unique individuals and as human beings. Like X-ray films on which the bones are the most distinct, because they are the strongest and most indestructible elements of the body, so it is that adversity reveals the eternal, and thus indestructible, qualities of the soul.

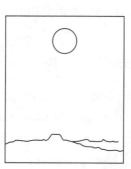

2

THE GROUND GIVES WAY UNDER US

W̲hen there is a *before* and an *after*, when there is an event that marks the moment that brings ordinary life to an end, which is often the case with medical conditions, the shift that occurs has the force of a natural disaster, a personal earthquake that disturbs the ground under us. Before the diagnosis, before the operation, before the accident, before the discovery that there is something wrong, we live in innocence or denial. Then everything changes, and we feel that nothing may ever be the same again.

In this, we may feel like Persephone,[1] the maiden in Greek mythology who was gathering flowers in the meadow when the earth opened up in front of her, and out of the deepest, darkest vent in the earth came Hades, the Lord of the Underworld, in his black chariot drawn by black horses, to abduct her. He pulled Persephone to him, and she screamed in fear as they circled the field, and then horses and chariot, carrying

1. For a further version of the myth, Jean Shinoda Bolen, *Demeter and Persephone: The Abduction into the Underworld* (Boulder, Colo.: Sounds True Recordings, 1992), audiotape.

Hades, and the terrified Persephone, plunged back from where they came, and the earth closed over as if nothing had happened.

Encounter with Hades: Loss and Vulnerability

One moment, Persephone had nothing more on her mind than which beautiful flower to pick; the sky was blue, the sun was warm, and all was well. The next moment, she was in the underworld and nothing was the same as before. Her innocence and security were violated; she was helpless and at the mercy of forces beyond her previous knowledge. This myth applies to everyone. *Persephone* is the innocent part of men and women, youngsters and elders, who encounter *Hades* as the perpetrator of incest, rape, mugging, betrayal, of any unexpected and unforeseen act that shocks us into an awareness of our emotional or physical vulnerability. Hades is also the symbolic event that exposes us to a specific awareness of good and evil. Before Hades, we feel protected; after Hades we know that we are not. Once a laboratory test comes back HIV+ or a biopsy reveals cancer, through whatever means we learn of a life-threatening illness, the effect is the same: *Persephone*—the assumption of youth and health, the assumption of safety and immunity from disease and death—has been violated and taken into the underworld.

For many of us, poetic metaphor expresses our feelings and is a means through which we communicate our perceptions and understand the meaning of an experience. *Illness as a descent of the soul into the underworld* is a metaphor that brings to the intuitive mind and knowing heart a depth of understanding that cannot be grasped consciously otherwise. It is also in the language of the soul.

The Underworld of Fear

When the possibility or reality of a major medical illness arises, when we or someone we love are to be hospitalized for observation, diagnosis, or treatment, it is metaphorically like being abducted into the underworld—that subconscious or unconscious realm—where we are assailed by fears and vulnerabilities that we usually keep buried there and at a distance: we may be exposed to fear of death, fear of pain, of dismemberment, dependency, disfigurement, dementia, and depression. The possibility of becoming seriously sick or impaired exposes us to fears and realities to do with the loss of relationships, of work, of manhood or womanhood, of opportunities and dreams; we fear being a burden, financial and otherwise; we fear for our children or others who depend upon us; we fear that we may no longer be ourselves, and those fears are sometimes compounded by how others treat us or how we react when childhood insecurities become entwined with present-day adult anxieties. We can lose the best of ourselves in sinkholes of self-pity, or become mired obsessively in "Why me?"

Sick or potentially sick people are often infantilized, women especially. Doctors and others often talk about us as if we were not there. If we make a fuss, we are not being good patients. Everyone is concerned with the medical problem, not with the psyche: the message a patient gets is to keep your fears to yourself and put on a good face; *be a good girl* or *act like a man,* and do what the doctor says. You are not to be angry. You are not to question authority. You are now in the underworld of your fears but are not to mention it. If you are angry or self-pitying, if you become emotional, if you want doctors or nurses to pay attention to your feelings, you are being a problem. Attending to emotions takes time, and when there is just so much time to do hospital rounds, or so much time allotted to see each patient, a patient or a relative who needs or wants reassurance or further explanations is often seen as demanding or even as requiring a psychiatric consultation.

The Underworld of Depression

The underworld can also be a state of mind that resembles the realm of Hades in which abducted Persephone was an imprisoned captive. It was a dim world inhabited by the shades of the dead, which were recogniz-able but without substance, bloodless images like holograms or like memories devoid of emotion. This is the realm of depression when we are cut off from our feelings, which illness and the effort to repress all feelings and fears can bring us into. We then act as if we were inani-mate, obedient, cooperative objects. The diagnosis of a life-threatening illness and the need to respond immediately to medical advice about what to do invites us to dissociate from our feelings. Whether from depression or from dissociation, the result is often the same. Detached from emotions, a person can then be the picture of the good patient who enters the hospital as if it were a body repair shop.

The Underworld of the Soul

The underworld is also a soul realm, a place of great inner richness. This is the realm of Pluto—the Latin name for Hades—which means riches or treasures underground. This is the psychological layer that contains the potentials we have not developed, the talents and inclinations that once mattered to us, the emotions we hid from view and then lost touch with. Beyond this personal level lies the richness of the archetypal or sym-bolic layer of the collective unconscious, where patterns, instincts, all that is human resides, a deep core of meaning that dreams and creativity draw from. Here are the wellsprings of the soul, the spiritual instinct that directs us toward divinity in the same unconscious way that flowers turn to face the sun. Here the psychological quest for wholeness and meaning begins. Here in the archetypal realm, death and rebirth are metaphors, and the reality of physical death, which may be terrifying to the ego, is countered by dreams which have an entirely different perspective.

We can enter into this soul realm by musing upon the symbols, themes, and possible meaning of dreams that we record and remem-ber; by following impulses to play music, sing, or listen to music; to dance, paint, or draw; to honor and express what comes up when we are open to our own flow of feelings; to keep a journal; to write poetry; through prayer and meditation, to be in silence or conversation at a soul level. When these gateways to the soul realm are familiar, access is not difficult.

This inner world of the soul is a foreign country for many. The extroverted person who prides himself or herself on being practical and logical, the caretakers who focus on the needs of others, the work-oriented, for whom being productive is a measure of their worth, often have not ventured into their inner world very much. The resources of the inner world that can be tapped to help heal body and soul then need to be learned—which later chapters focus upon. To learn of the potential riches of this aspect of the underworld, to want firsthand knowledge, and be willing to spend energy and time to get there, is the beginning; keeping a log—on paper, in memory—is a next step, out of which comes the value to oneself of attending to images, phrases, of feelings and thoughts that emerge out of one's own depths. A vivid dream needs to be attended to by writing it down; it will not likely be remembered otherwise, and even if remembered, details will be lost. Paying attention to the details of the dream may lead to musing upon parts of it, which leads to further memories and associations. It may move a person who otherwise might be either unfocused or focused on discomfort, or focused obsessively, to become absorbed in a communication from the dreaming psyche. To muse induces a meditative attitude, which is an open, receptive mind and heart. This is what solitude, meditation, or being receptive in prayer does for some of us. This is what backpacking, running, fishing, gardening, or sewing does for others. Whatever it takes for us to hear the small still voice within, or reach the still point at the center, are the means, the access to the inner world of soul. When this realm is unknown terrain, or when illness makes ways we once used no longer possible, we can try ways that have worked for others, or learn from others. Just as one seeks a referral to a doctor and checks on credentials, experience, and affiliations, so is it possible to seek counseling or classes on various means of meditation, spiritual development, dream and journal work, and expressive therapies.

The Underworld of the Spirits

Life-endangering illness can have the effect of thinning the veils between this world and the otherworld of the spirits. People tell me such things as having had vivid, distinctly remembered conversations with figures they clearly saw and yet knew were not part of their ordinary reality, or of feeling the comforting presence of people who had died even though they neither heard nor saw them, or of telepathically communicating with an otherworldly figure when they were gravely ill. Less common and more dramatic are the stories told by people who were near death when they met otherworld figures who told them that it was not their time. Twice now, women have told me of having an old, apparently Native American woman appear to them when they failed to respond to medical treatment and were dying; her appearance was an intervention that changed the course of the illness. One of them had a fever of unknown origin that broke, only then. The other knew, as a result of this visitation or vision, that she was misdiagnosed, and efforts on her part led to a correct diagnosis of Lyme disease and proper treatment. Both women recovered and in their respective ways, became involved in bringing alternative medicine into more mainstream awareness. Illness brought them close to death and a nonordinary reality, which was both a turning point for the illness and the inspiration to help others after getting well.

At his memorial service, Gary Walsh, a San Francisco therapist turned activist, who organized the first candlelight AIDS march and debated Jesse Helms on AIDS, was vividly present on film. In a videotaped interview done a few days before his death from AIDS, he told us about being visited twice by a man whom many in the audience had known, a man who had recently died. While Gary was physically wasted in appearance, he was assertive, clear, and utterly convincing. He asserted that he was not asleep and that he was not hallucinating when this man appeared in his room and told him not to worry, that he would be there when Gary died and crossed over. Gary demanded in a prove-it-to-me tone, that he appear to him one more time. A couple of days later, again when he was awake and mentally clear, this man appeared again, very briefly and impatient, reiterating that he would be there when Gary died, and obviously put out at having to make this extra visit, because he "had other things to do."

Descending in Stages into the Underworld: The Inanna Myth

The descent of the soul into the underworld which illness can precipitate, does not always have the impact of a shocking, sudden, and unexpected abduction or the immediate devastation of being at the center of a major earthquake. Persephone's myth applies when this is so, but there is a second myth that parallels the experience of people whose illness and descent occurs in stages through an incremental loss of footing in the ordinary world of good health: either they have an illness with a gradually worsening pattern, or they maintain the illusion of being in control and minimize the emotional impact of having a serious medical problem. The myth that resembles the journey they take goes back at least five thousand years to the Sumerian goddess Inanna.[2]

Inanna was the Queen of Heaven and Earth. Heeding the news that her sister goddess Ereshkigal, Queen of the Underworld, was suffering and in pain, she decided to pay her a visit. Inanna mistakenly assumed that she could descend with ease. She would find however, that the power and authority she had in the upperworld had no bearing on how she would be treated in the underworld.

Inanna knocked imperiously on the gate to the underworld, demanding that the door be opened. The gatekeeper asked who she was, and then told her that in order to pass through, there was a price. She would find that there was not just one gate, but seven. At each one, the gatekeeper told her that she must take off something she was wearing to pass through. Each time, Inanna responded indignantly, shocked

2. Refer to Diane Wolkstein and Samuel Noah Kramer, *Inanna: Queen of Heaven and Earth* (New York: Harper & Row, 1983), pp. 52–71.

that this should be so, with the words: "What *is* this?" Each time, she was told: "Quiet, Inanna, the ways of the underworld are perfect. They may not be questioned."

Her magnificent headdress, the crown that designated her authority, was removed at the first gate. The lapis necklace was taken from her neck at the second gate, the double strand of rich beads was removed from her breasts at the third gate. She was stripped of her breastplate at the fourth gate, of her gold bracelet at the fifth gate. The lapis measuring rod and line were taken from her at the sixth gate. At the seventh gate, she was stripped of her royal robe. Naked and bowed low, she entered the underworld.

Over and over, at each gate, symbols of power, prestige, wealth, and office were taken from her. Over and over, at each gate, the removal of something else that covered her, was unexpected. Over and over, she would say, "What is this?" and be told, "Quiet, Inanna. The rules of the underworld are perfect. They may not be questioned."

Whenever a person becomes a patient and enters a hospital, the experience is not unlike Inanna's. Metaphorically, there are a series of gates to go through, and at each one, something is taken away. At the door to the hospital, he or she unwittingly crosses through the first gate. In increments, thereafter, a patient is stripped of dignity, choice, and authority. However important the patient is in the world, however significant he or she is to someone else does not matter here.

The second gate is the admissions desk, where each person must sign a number of papers in order to be admitted, receives a hospital number, has a plastic identification band fastened around a wrist, and may be given a receipt in return for surrendering valuables.

The third gate is usually the hospital room. Here each patient takes off street clothes which are reflections of individuality and status and puts on the standard hospital gown that often is ill-fitting, too short, and open up the back. Then there are the other gates, through which a patient is taken on a gurney or in a wheelchair, to radiology for X-rays or more sophisticated tests, to other specialized rooms for blood tests unknown, fearful world, patients feel metaphorically left hanging on a hook awaiting news that they can come back to life.

In the bowels of the hospital, or the receding world that illness creates, or in the fearful half-light of the psychological underworld, patients enter the realm of Ereshkigal, when they reach the point of realizing that their old self and old life are dead, at least for now, perhaps forever. For the soul, this can be a turning point: facing the possibility of disability or death can be reorienting, it can bring about a massive change in priorities, and bring to the forefront questions of meaning and meaninglessness about how we are living our lives, about what really matters, and whether we matter. For the ego that had maintained the illusion of control over fate, this is often the lowest point. For the person, if ego turns to soul to lead the way through the underworld, there will be unexpected discoveries. For *it's not what happens to us, but how we respond that ultimately matters* and shapes who we are from inside out.

Responding to Unchosen Circumstances

Ever since I read Viktor Frankl's book *Man's Search for Meaning,*[3] I have had an appreciation of a spiritual and psychological reality: that no matter how little control we may have over circumstances, even in the most terrible situation, we have a choice of how we will respond. This insight is empowering. Frankl and all of his relatives were taken into German concentration camps, where every one of his family members perished. In this situation, there was no freedom, no choice about what or whether one would eat or work or be sent to the gas chambers the next day. The prisoners were starved and beaten, their legs became swollen with edema; they were stripped of identity, reduced to a number, and denied basic human dignity. And yet, even here, there were choices to be made at a soul level. Some people just gave up; others

3. All references to Viktor Frankl are taken from Viktor E. Frankl, *Man's Search for Meaning: An Introduction to Logotherapy,* trans. Ilse Lasch (New York: Pocket Books, 1963).

or to have various scopes inserted into orifices or through body walls in order for the doctor to see inside the body.

When surgery is called for, the patient passes through more gates, to the preoperative area, into surgery, then into postoperative or intensive care, and in going through these particular gates loses both consciousness and usually a part of the body as well.

In coming to terms with having a life-threatening illness, a person often is stripped of emotional defenses as well. Denial, intellectualization, and rationalization may go, exposing a person to the painful realities of their lives as well of this illness. Addictions that kept feelings at a distance are taken away. People who use work and activity, alcohol or drugs to numb their feelings no longer can do this (though television, which may be the commonest addiction, is immediately turned on at many hospital bedsides).

When psychological defenses dissolve in the context of life-threatening illnesses, a descent into the underworld of depression and fear can occur. A dissolution of defenses against knowing the truth may reveal an emotionally and spiritually barren life, an empty marriage, or a meaningless job, as well as the reality of the seriousness of the medical condition and accompanying fears.

Metaphorically and actually, illness and hospitalizations strip us of what covered and protected us in many ways. Indignities happen, and a "What is this?" protest may be met by words and attitudes from hospital staff that resemble those that Inanna heard: "Quiet, Patient. The orders of the doctor are perfect. They may not be questioned." Even when our physicians are healers whom we trust, and they as well as the others communicate what and why whatever is being done is required, and even if we are fully involved in the decision making, the journey is still similar to Inanna's. There are still gates we go through, which strip us of persona and defense: we become exposed and bare-souled.

This stripping away makes it possible for us to reach depths within ourselves that we otherwise might not reach, where whatever we consigned there or abandoned or forgot of ourselves, suffers the pain of not being remembered or of not being integrated into our conscious personality or allowed expression. In remembering, we find ourselves connecting with soul. What is actively sought in a depth analysis may be inadvertently revealed as a result of having a disabling physical illness or entering a hospital with a condition that will take a patient through a difficult and uncertain course, through making a descent into the underworld. Psychological depth is the realm of Ereshkigal, as is death. When death takes on a reality and becomes close, soul questions arise.

The Underworld of Shadow and Depth: Ereshkigal's Realm

As Inanna can symbolize our upper, outer, or in-the-world personality, the part of us who is somebody in the world, so can Ereshkigal represent our unseen aspects and memories that we have kept hidden, in the shadow or innerworld; Ereshkigal can be a symbol of the cause of our suffering that we have ignored or depreciated and can only approach, humbled and made vulnerable by adversity. Ereshkigal is unattended when we deny whatever is personally meaningful and authentically true for us and are walled off from this *gnosis* or felt-knowledge. Going through the gates to our feelings and fears occurs when we incrementally go through layers of resistance to accepting the reality of illness.

People also make a descent with Inanna when they have gradually disabling illnesses, chronically worsening mental or physical health, illnesses that fall into a diagnostic limbo between the body and the psyche—environmental allergies, chronic fatigue syndrome, and psychosomatic illnesses—or have infectious or hereditary diseases that involve multiple systems and are progressive. The descent may take years, with the onset of a new set of symptoms, subsequent tests, and the prescriptions and procedures, like another gate to pass through.

Chemotherapy and radiation patients make an Inanna descent. Each treatment is another gate. After the second or third chemotherapy treatment, hair often falls out in clumps. On this descent at this gate, you surrender your head of hair, and even if you were expecting it, this

is a shock. For women especially, it is a loss that strikes at identit[y,] femininity. It is often a low point, a depressing time. The face i[n the] mirror is unfamiliar. "Who is this?"

Inanna was naked and bowed low when she entered the underw[orld;] she had been humbled and stripped as she descended, but the o[rdeal] was not yet over. When Inanna came into Ereshkigal's presence[, the] goddess of the underworld was not happy to see her. Filled with v[enom] and judgment, Ereshkigal gazed at Inanna with the baleful ey[es of] death and struck her dead. Then Inanna's body was hung on a h[ook,] where after three days, it began to decompose or turn into a sla[b of] green meat.

Inanna and Jesus: Transformation of Suffering

Inanna's fate at this point reminds me of Jesus, and the series of bet[ray]als, humiliations, and punishments he suffered on the way to the c[ross,] and as he hung from it on Good Friday until he was dead; his body [was] put in a tomb, hers hung on a hook for three days. When illness stri[kes,] people do feel betrayed and humiliated by their bodies, and pain is p[ain,] whether from a whip or being nailed to a cross or from some sou[rce] beneath our flesh. In the midst of suffering, many people feel like Jes[us,] alone and in pain, on the cross crying out, "My God, my God, w[hy] have you forsaken me?"

Just as hanging on the cross was not the end of Jesus's story, hang[ing] on a hook was not the end of Inanna and her myth. She too w[as] brought back to life, significantly transformed. In the language of t[he] soul, death is a major, recurring metaphor. On the spiritual journ[ey,] death of the old personality is required for an initiation, transform[a]tion, rebirth, or resurrection. On the medical journey, patients oft[en] feel like Inanna: the hospital feels like an underworld in which they a[re] stripped and humbled, and then unconscious under anesthesia, th[ey] literally become a slab of meat on an operating table. Or after a seri[es] of tests and treatments, each of which takes them deeper into a

acted in the same inhuman way as their captors toward weaker inmates; and still others shared what they had, maintained loyalties, and even sacrificed themselves so other prisoners might survive longer. In this apparently meaningless and inhuman existence, Frankl noted that there remained a choice of attitude to take. He emphasized that the search for meaning is essential, and that the will to live depended upon it. If suffering or dying is the task, doing it well or poorly is a choice.

Several years ago, I met with the nursing staff of a general hospital unit following two deaths that occurred within days of each other. They were in grief and in guilt, and needed help with feelings stirred up by these deaths. Both patients were men who had died of AIDS. One of them was someone that the staff had come to know well and love, over years of multiple hospitalizations. They admired his courage as they helped him through his relapses, and with a posthospital follow-up program, maintained contact with him during remissions. They were emotionally as well as professionally invested in his struggle. His death was mercifully peaceful and a personal loss to most of them. Their reaction to him grew out of his response to having AIDS: like a man dealt a bad hand but playing it well, he put his energy into living as fully and as long as he could.

The other man was characterized as the most disliked patient any of them could remember. Efforts to help him were met with profanity, kindness was ridiculed and thrown back in their faces sarcastically. He was uncooperative, unappreciative, and full of hate. Bitterness, rage, and resentment was his response to having AIDS. He upset and disturbed other patients. He made it difficult to put in IVs or draw blood, and as he wished AIDS on others, contamination by his blood was a frightening possibility. Nurses came to hate him and dreaded the next incident he would provoke. Some found themselves wishing he would die. Their negative feelings were so at odds with their intellectual grasp of why he was behaving this way and their sense of themselves as good people and professionals, that when he died, alone with no one who mourned him, they were filled with guilt and shame. Both men shaped the last part of their lives by how they responded to having AIDS and how they treated the people around them. The legacy of feelings that they left behind grew directly out of these choices.

The choice of how we respond to what happens to us usually remains, no matter how difficult the course. When we lose this choice is difficult to determine, because even when there is mental clouding, character seems to remain and influence response. It is not just circumstance that shapes us, either. Adults who have retained the capacity to love and hope and have faith and did not become like the people who abused them in childhood, somehow drew upon an inner wisdom, and chose not to do to others what was done to them, or give up on themselves or on people, or succumb to hopelessness or cynicism and self-pity, choices that others in similar circumstances have made that diminish spirit and soul. Variations of these same choices of how we will respond and what we will become as a result, present themselves over and over to all of us in life. If our character and development of soul is shaped by us over time in much the same way as clay is worked upon before it must go through the fire, then we are both the artist and the work itself. We are a work in progress until the final touch. How we respond when we suffer unfairly shapes us, and what we do when we know we are dying makes a difference if we truly are spiritual beings on a human path.

Living in the Shadow of Death

The epidemic of AIDS and cancer, especially cancer of the breast for women, has been called a holocaust. We hear that one out of eight women will get cancer of the breast, or one out of three people will get cancer in their lifetime. For gay men, the impact of numbers is staggering and personal, not statistical. To have a circle of friends and a community more than decimated by AIDS, an address book with lines drawn through the names of men who have died on every page, and an awareness that the living who are HIV+ will die, is to be in a personal holocaust.

Appearances make the parallels graphic. Patients with either progressive disease or those in the throes of aggressive chemotherapy or radiation therapy often lose appetite and weight. They can begin to resemble inmates of concentration camps, where Viktor Frankl learned about choice and survival of spirit in the midst of pain, deprivation, malnourishment, and suffering. Between the illness itself and treatment, there is almost always pain and suffering. There are times when food cannot be kept down, or cannot be absorbed. Malnourishment is common. While there are no barbed fences, the necessity of being in a hospital linked to an intravenous bottle is as confining. In a hospital as in the concentration camps, people live in a valley of the shadow of death, susceptible to feeling powerless and in danger of giving up.

On AIDS units and in the radiation therapy waiting areas, patients become aware that they are not alone in their suffering, that they are not the only one. Just as Frankl noted the way inmates responded, similar observations can be made in hospital settings. One such observer, Phil Head, a contributor to a series of essays in *When the Worst That Can Happen Already Has,* described what he saw. "You watch the ones who sadly give up. They don't walk into the room and say, 'I give up, I have cancer,' but in the way they accept the treatments and the way they relate to the other people, you know they've given up. . . .Then there are the people who try, to the best of their abilities, to spread a little fellowship and humor. From the very beginning, humor for me was a big help. As long as I was able to laugh at myself, the treatments, and my circumstances, there was hope."[4]

Humor is an expression of spirit and fellowship in the midst of a descent into the underworld, it's a means of commenting on reality and getting through uncertain times of risk and pain. (Frankl described humor at Auschwitz and Dachau as among "the soul's weapons in the fight for self-preservation.") When one has been stripped of the outer garments of dignity and there is no visible means of security, humor

4. Phil Head, "I Immediately Took Action," in Dennis Wholey, ed., *When the Worst That Can Happen Already Has* (New York: Hyperion Press, 1992), p. 159.

comes from soul's perspective and laughter changes our biochemistry and psychology.

While humor may seem irreverent and far removed from a five-thousand-year-old goddess myth or the two-thousand-year-old Easter story, myth and humor have much in common in helping us through a period in the underworld. Both feed the spirit, and are expressions of the unconquerable element in us. Humor and myth provide perspective on our suffering and make pain easier to bear. Each also is a commentary on there being something more to what is going on than meets the eye.

Entry to the Underworld: Ready or Not

There are many good reasons for an immediate admission to the hospital, such as traumatic injuries from accidents or violence, severe burns, a likely myocardial infarct, hemorrhaging, being unconscious, having a raging fever—any state in which immediate care could make the difference between life and death. At Los Angeles General County Hospital, where I interned, anyone who arrived in a critical condition was called "a red blanket." The patient was immediately put on a gurney, a red blanket (in actuality, a bright red sheet) was thrown over him, and an attendant wheeled the gurney on a nonstop elevator to an admitting ward. When a red blanket arrived on the floor, that patient was seen immediately.

In contrast, many people go to a doctor's office with symptoms that have been present for a while, often after having had to wait for days or even weeks for this appointment, and are told that they must go from the office to the hospital immediately. In an atmosphere of fear and urgency, there is then no time to prepare others, or get some matters settled that might otherwise be major worries, or get a second opinion, or be able to inquire into alternatives, or become psychologically and spiritually supported and prepared for an undertaking that will tax the body and soul of the patient. Doctors who instill fear, don't discuss options, and take immediate charge under noncritical conditions usually render the patient helpless to chart his or her own course. Fear of malpractice suits, unfamiliarity with the patient as a person, the economics of insurance coverage, may make this course the prudent one for the physician, and a very difficult situation for the patient to resist.

This is a critical moment. The decision to be immediately admitted to the hospital may be the right one, and you may be relieved that this is happening, because you have had a feeling that something quite serious was not being attended to, and now it is. You may intuitively trust the doctor and the decision. Or, as is sometimes the case, there may be an inner resistance, an intuition or feeling that you need more information, or need to sort out the situation, or need to take care of other matters before you can go in. For the soul, and quite possibly for the body, it matters whether *you* are ready or not. For you are not just being admitted to the hospital, you are on a soul journey that will take you into the underworld.

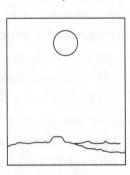

3

HARBINGER OF TRUTH

A serious illness takes us into a time which is both strange and scary for almost everyone. It is a life-changing, major event that brings the possibility of death or disability close to us. "Biting the bullet"—that western frontier expression to do with submitting to surgery that absolutely must be done with no available anesthesia, and biting down rather than crying out—is now what is called for metaphorically. It means having the courage to face the reality or possibility of having an illness that may kill you. It means suffering pain that goes with the disease or the apprehension of it. It means enduring the treatment. What ails the body is at the immediate forefront, but attending to what ails the soul and is not right with our lives is often not far behind. Any serious medical condition—a heart attack, a bleeding ulcer, malignant hypertension, a malignancy—may have an impact on the psyche by cutting through layers of denial. An illness may confront us with what we know in our bones about being unhappy or self-destructive and have thus far disregarded or denied. Biting the bullet then applies to more than the medical problem; it's facing what is wrong with other aspects of our lives and what must be done. Once we face a medical truth and submit to what must be done to survive, barriers to other truths often come down as well. When this is so, it is a harbinger of change that will come next on the soul level.

When an illness is life-threatening, we are usually able to recognize how insignificant and unimportant many of our everyday concerns are. We may find that we are, for this time, free of neurotic preoccupations; what matters, for a change, may be what *really* matters. "Cancer can be an instant cure for neurosis" was how several women at a conference for breast cancer survivors put it.

At this same meeting, women who had made major changes in their lives as a result of a cancer diagnosis and were not just surviving the cancer but thriving remarked how their illness was "the worst thing that had ever happened to them *and* the best thing that had happened to them." Men who were work-driven, aggressive, and ambitious until they were felled by heart attacks, who slowed down and refocused, say the same thing. Usually these women and men took a good, long look at what was wrong in their lives, and acted decisively to end what was bad for them—at the body and soul level—and moved toward what sustained and nourished them, also at the body and soul level.

It may be that they (finally) ended dysfunctional, soul-draining relationships with narcissistic, controlling, needy, abusive, or chronically angry people, who responded in their characteristically self-absorbed fashion to the news of the life-threatening illness. Or they (finally) stopped self-destructive additions to cigarettes, alcohol, or work. Usually, they (finally) acted on their own best behalf because they knew that their life depended upon it. In this, their illness served as a wake-up call that enabled them to face what they had resisted.

Enacting the Psyche Myth: Illness and Soul Growth

In the Greek myth of Eros and Psyche[1] (Love and Soul), Psyche's story is about the growth of the soul that began with her decision to face the

---

1. Paraphrased from Jean Shinoda Bolen, *The Myth of Eros and Psyche* (Boulder, Colo.: Sounds True Recordings, 1992), audiotape.

truth, and led to her being on her own, challenged to complete tasks that were initially beyond her ability to perform. In the myth, her unseen bridegroom would come to her in the dark of the night and be gone by morning. Metaphorically, she was in an unconscious relationship. Fearing that he could be a monster, Psyche followed her sisters' advice, hid a lamp and a knife, and waited until he had fallen asleep. She needed the lamp to see him, and the knife to cut off his head if indeed he were a monster.

The Lamp and the Knife

These two symbols, the lamp and the knife, are both necessary for a psyche—for a soul—to act decisively when we know the truth. The lamp is a symbol of illumination, of consciousness, the means of seeing a situation clearly. The knife, like the sword, is a symbol of decisive action, of the capacity to cut through confusion, to sever bonds when necessary. The lamp without the knife is not adequate: it is insight into the situation without the capacity to act upon this perception. Usually if we cannot act upon what we know, clarity dims—it's too uncomfortable to be aware; adaptation, rationalization, and denial work against staying conscious.

That her life could depend upon severing bonds with several people who depleted her was an intuition heeded by one woman who, on getting a diagnosis of cancer, met with each one to tell them of her diagnosis and with tact and nonnegotiable clarity say that she would no longer be available for phone conversations or time together. For another woman, once she learned her diagnosis, it became possible to distance herself from her narcissistic mother and to weather the guilt and accusations that accompanied it. That her life depended upon divorcing her husband was made clear to a third woman, who for the first and only time in her life heard an emphatic voice in her head say, "You *must* get a divorce." This, when she was in her doctor's office to hear the results of a biopsy that confirmed that she had cancer.

Insight followed by decisive action—the lamp and the sword—are needed for people to change or end difficult, damaging, or destructive relationships. Before the diagnosis, many of these women had the lamp but not the sword; they knew that they were in relationships that took a toll of them, but did not feel entitled to act upon this knowledge. Women are often held captive by the emotional needs or intimidating demands of others, coupled with an inability to say "No!" These people are draining, they take from us; there is a cost in emotional and physical resources, in time and energy. Resentment grows when we know this but do not speak up and act to change or end these relationships. Continuing to be in them has a depressing effect on our mood and well-being, which in turn can depress our immune system and reduce our resistance to disease.

Inner Wisdom

There are crucial times when health or death are held in delicate balance and could be tipped in either direction. It is at these times that heeding what the soul knows or the body needs may make all the difference. There is an inner wisdom that knows such matters, which comes through to us as strong intuitions, as *gnosis* or felt-knowledge, as an interior certainly beyond logic, or even as an audible voice; it is what we know in our bones.

Myths and symbols are in the language of the soul. A myth helps us to take a situation to heart and know what we must do: if it is to see the truth and act upon it, then the image of Psyche with her lamp and knife provides a mythic perspective. A symbolic object can then be a talisman that helps us do what we need to do. For example, I have a beautifully crafted sword with a silver hilt and a clear crystal shaft that is only about two inches long. I can hold it in the palm of my hand and mentally review what it symbolizes and then take it with me into a situation where I need to call upon those very qualities. When I gave a similar sword to my friend to carry with her, it came with my support for what she needed to do. When a symbol is presented with words that convey the intention of the gift, the moment and the object are imbued with ritual significance. Like passing a literal torch, these are rituals that empower us by infusing an act with a deeper meaning. To think and act this way is magical, metaphoric thinking that can call forth the qualities we need from within ourselves and may also tap into sources of help that lie beyond us, as prayer does.

The Need to Say "No!"

In the myth, Psyche's final task involved making a descent into the underworld and returning. She carried a cake in each hand for Cerberus, the three-headed, terrible hound, one to give him to let her pass through the gates into the realm of Hades, the second to give him when she left. She brought coins for Charon the ferryman, the fare to take and return her across the river Styx. And she was told that she would be asked for help that she must not give. Instead, she must harden her heart to pity, say "No" and go on. Three times, she heard pleas to help: a lame old man with a lame donkey asked her to pick up a few twigs that had dropped from the donkey's load; then a dead man who lacked a coin for the ferryman and was floating in the river Styx raised his hands for her to grasp, beseeching her to help him cross; and finally, three dim-sighted old women asked her to stop and help them with their weaving. Three times, we imagine that she felt pulled toward helping, but each time she heeded the advice she was given, hardened her heart to pity, said "No" and walked on.

Had she stopped to lend a hand, she would have had to let go of the cake she carried in that hand. Though it seemed a small thing to lose, without it she would never again see the light of day. For without that second cake, she could not placate the terrible three-headed dog and could not leave the underworld. If she had been unable to say "No," she would have lost what she needed to make the journey and return.

When we are seriously ill or recovering from surgery, radiation, chemotherapy, or any life-threatening or health-threatening condition, we are in the underworld. Or we may be accompanying someone we love through the underworld, and need all the resources we have for the both of us. The need to conserve our strength, to not extend ourselves at such times, is advice we need to heed. The Psyche myth may make the point in a deeper way than a rational explanation, especially when—as is often the case—people who drain and deplete us, have held us in the relationship through guilt and the assumption that we are responsible for them.

Moments of Truth

When we are going through an underworld phase, there is the possibility that we will not return if we do not hold on to what we need. When this part of the Psyche myth strikes a note, we know that the difference between making our way back to physical, psychological, or spiritual health may hinge upon very little. Like Psyche, we may be asked to do something that seems on the surface a small expenditure of time and energy, and we may be drawn to help, out of compassion and because we feel mean-spirited and selfish (guilty) if we say "No." *It is not a small thing; it is a moment of truth.* To hold on to the message of the myth when we know it is true (and yet have trouble justifying it to others) may be possible if we imagine we are Psyche making a descent into the underworld and our return depends on whether we can harden our heart to pity and guilt and say "No" to whatever and whoever we know will drag our spirit down and take energy and optimism from us that we cannot afford to lose.

Taking Psyche's Story to Heart

I have told the story of Psyche in the underworld many, many times and know how powerful the story is when a listener has an Aha! recognition of its personal meaning. Three times, Psyche—whose name means "Soul"—was tested: will she say "No" and hold on to what she needs to make it through this part of her life, when the outcome of the rest of her life depends upon it? Many listeners, especially women with selfish parents, partners, or others with narcissistic needs, immediately identify with this part of the myth and know that it applies to their lives, right now.

When we recognize that these symbolic figures may also be representations of "who" we need to say "No" to *in ourselves,* Psyche's story takes us to yet a level deeper. Do we need to say "No" to the parts of ourselves that are in some way lame, dim-sighted, or a drag on us? A life-threatening illness takes us into the underworld, where life as well as soul is at risk. Insights may make a crucial difference. Look to this myth: survival may depend upon saying "No" to self-pity or to a tendency to weave worst-case outcomes or to taking on burdens that belong to someone else.

I have found that once we have clarity to know what is right for us and what is wrong for us, we are invariably tested to see if we really got the lesson. Circumstances and individuals present themselves: Will we recognize that this is another version of the same pattern or person that has been destructive to us before? Will we stand tall and say "No!" this time around? Once we pass by the temptation as many times as we seem to need to in order to be out of danger of succumbing, the psychological terrain and the emotional weather change. We find ourselves in a new phase of our lives and are able to say "Yes!" wholeheartedly, often for the very first time, because we have come to know what we feel, trust our perceptions, and can count on ourselves. There is a need to be able to say "No" that precedes a genuine "Yes," when our actions have previously been determined by compliance, conformity, or fear of the reaction of others.

When a story such as Psyche's is taken to heart, a person sees herself or himself as the protagonist in a version of the same story. It can be a force for change, if a myth provides the means to see what is happening, inspires us, and gives us strength to act. The power of a myth lies in the application of it to real life. Personal stories have the same power to affect us, if we can identify with the situation and with the person.

Discriminating Actions

If you are in a hospital or at home recovering, still tiring easily and needing all the energy you can muster for your recovery, the opportunity to take the message of the myth to heart and act upon it may apply to visitors and calls. When I think of visiting hours in hospitals, I am reminded of Anne Morrow Lindbergh's observation in *Gift from the Sea*: "The most exhausting thing in life, I have discovered, is being insincere."[2] For both visitors and patients, bedside visits can be tiring and trying. Patients often find themselves needing to reassure their healthy callers that they are fine or will be fine, when they have doubts and fears; or they hear how fine they look when they know it's not true. Patients can be captive audiences, as visitors chatter, tell medical horror stories, or overstay visits. Then there are relatives who seem to be news-gatherers, often indistinguishable from bearers of bad tidings, as they pass on stories. Obligatory visits made by well-mannered people are another category. In the midst of a life-threatening illness, a patient may be in a personal underworld and yet be playing the part of a gracious hostess.

To be like Psyche in this situation means saying "No" at many levels and recognizing the importance of doing so—to hold that symbolic lamp and knife again, to see clearly and take appropriate action. Bedside phones can be disconnected while one sleeps or is not up to receiving calls. Hospitals can let people know that you are not receiving visitors or that visiting time is restricted, which is appropriate medically in intensive care units and other circumstances. Visitors can be limited and therefore selected. However, with convalescence, rehabilitation, in ongoing treatment, or in remission, there are further decisions that may

2. Anne Morrow Lindbergh, *Gift from the Sea*, 20th anniversary ed. (New York: Pantheon, 1975), p. 32.

need to be made because visits from others can help or hinder our efforts to become well.

A clergywoman receiving chemotherapy for cancer comes to my mind. Since she had many friends and a large congregation, there were numerous visitors. In her pastoral role, she was the comforter, and even though she was the patient, both she and others would fall into the old pattern; she found herself ministering to their concerns for her and hearing about what was going on in their lives. It was draining. While she did not want to talk about herself much, she did not want to be isolated by saying "No" to having visitors, but something had to be done. With a discriminating heart to feel what was healing and helpful and what was not, she acted and the result was quite wonderful.

What she decided to do fit the needs of her personality and her situation beautifully. She valued her solitude, especially in the mornings, and did not have a knack for the easy sociability that might lift someone else's spirits. She had come to know members of her congregation and had counseled and prayed with them during their difficulties. While she did not want to talk about herself with them, she knew that praying together or being together at a soul level was mutually nourishing. Another consideration was her energy. Seeing more than one person at a time, long visits, or making small talk drained her. On the basis of such considerations, she let it be known what she needed, which was welcomed by people who cared about her.

Following her specific requests, she had mornings to herself. No one dropped in. People came in the afternoon for half an hour at the most, greeted her with a hug, had a cup of tea, and prayed in silence with her. They entered a peaceful room, she was prepared for them, and it was a loving and sacred time for both. Each day, it was usual for two people to come, usually separately and as scheduled—for the scheduling itself was part of her solution.

Hearing one woman's story evokes the possibility of doing the same: if she could do that, then what might you do? Her story has made me think about what I might do if I were recuperating or undergoing energy-depleting therapies. The idea of having to carry on insincerely with visitors while sick is more than I would bear. Instead of making small talk, which drains me, I might ask some of my visitors to read aloud from a book that I would enjoy hearing them read. I might ask some to hold my hand, and meditate or pray silently with me; like the clergywoman I also know how comforting and healing it is to be together in silence in prayer or meditation. If there was a particular part of my body in need of healing, I would have some visitors lay hands on that place, for I know that love is healing, and that people, animals, and plants grow and heal when touched. I would want to have beauty within sight, and have room for humor, laughter, touch, music, prayer—for soul.

What do *you* want? What would help heal you? Can you ask for it? Insist upon it? Can you say "No" to what or who depletes you, and bring what you need into your life? Might your actual life, and certainly the quality of it, depend upon choosing to do what nourishes your soul with your time and energy? If you are in the underworld of an illness, then you are in that part of the journey where the task is to say "No" to anything you do not want to do that takes a toll on your limited strength, "No" to anything you intuitively realize is wrong for you or wrong timing for you, to make decisions about which doctors and what treatments you will undergo. The ability to act as a warrior on your own behalf may begin with decisions about your visitors and extend from here into the whole of your life.

Warrior Marks

My image of what a hero looks like and what heroic means has been changed by watching ordinary people go through the ordeals that an illness and medical procedures take them through. Speaking before large groups of women survivors of cancer, seeing many with turbans covering their bald heads, or heads covered with fine downy hair from chemotherapy, knowing that most also bear surgical scars and some have radiation burns or bone-marrow-site scars, and that all of them have gone through or are in the midst of underworld descents, I have felt humbled by being in their presence. They are veterans, survivors, unrecognized heroes; the rest of us are civilians in comparison.

The only similarity for me was how I felt during my medical school and training years, especially in internship, with our thirty-six-hours-on, twelve-hours-off rotations; then it felt that we were in the front lines of life and death, while the rest of the world were civilians. Yet we were not at risk of becoming casualties, of being a statistic or a number in a body count.

Cancer patients and AIDS patients are like soldiers were in Vietnam: they are living through uncertainties and risks, they lose their friends to the enemy, perhaps even holding them in their arms as they die, they run into unexpected complications, and the appearance of new symptoms is the equivalent of being ambushed, stepping on mines, or being shot at by snipers. The enemy is near, deadly, and for the most part unseen. Patients, like soldiers in Vietnam, are caught up in a war that lasts for years, while contemporaries go on with their lives as usual. Just as many were blamed for participating in this war, there are patients who are blamed for having the disease, cancer as well as AIDS.

Meanwhile, women patients usually continue to hold down the home front as well. And just as men in foxholes got "Dear John" letters, so it seems that many women with cancer are emotionally abandoned or even left by husbands and lovers; on top of coping with cancer, they then also find themselves having to cope with the aftermath of ended marriages and relationships.

Often, abandonment occurred before the cancer, with depression and lack of reason to live depressing an immune system. When cancer arises, a patient who may have sometimes wished she were dead, now becomes confronted with the reality that she could be dead. For many, this mobilizes an inner warrior, and taps into a wish to live. The cancer then serves as a wake-up call to the importance of life, and in the process of coping with the cancer, the patient discovers strengths she never knew she had.

In this, a patient is like Psyche, a mythic figure whose psychology resembles many women who survive cancer. Psyche was an abandoned woman when she began the journey that called upon her to complete four tasks, each of which was beyond anything she had done before. Psyche's journey was not in response to "a call to adventure," which Joseph Campbell noted began the Hero's Journey. Nor did she resemble the archetypal hero, who is usually stronger and more advantaged than an ordinary mortal. Each new task seemed impossible at first. The difficulty initially overwhelmed Psyche, and then something (ants, a green reed, an eagle, a talking tower—symbols for the kind of inner strength or knowledge she needed) would come to her aid or give her advice that would enable her to find a way to complete the task and go on, stronger than before.

When adversity arises as a life-threatening illness, or calls upon a person to enter a hospital for major surgery, it is a heroic journey that is not respected as such, any more than the potentially life-threatening and always life-altering experience of pregnancy, labor, and delivery, which is also heroic, goes unrecognized as such. In both circumstances, people find fortitude, courage, the ability to endure pain, and strengths they never dreamed they ever had.

When my son, Andy, had to go through a series of major and minor operations, I saw his courage, character, and quiet strength emerge. Circumstances—his fate—required that he make a medical descent into the underworld, where he faced risk, pain, and uncertainty. The same month that he became twenty-one, Andy faced his most risky and difficult operation. He entered surgery to have a nonmalignant tumor removed that was unfortunately located in a dangerous place. It was pressing on his spinal cord in his neck, and had already displaced the cord slightly to one side. If it wasn't removed, it would result in a spinal cord compression. On the other hand, any mishap in surgery could result in serious damage to the spinal cord or the nerves that come off it. To reach the site, surgeons had to go through the bony vertebral bones of the spine, and then the dura and other finer protective coverings. Under the circumstances, surgery was not only risky, it was very long, and recovery from anesthesia and from the operation also took time, and was very uncomfortable. Because this surgery coincided with his becoming twenty-one, it made me think of the rites of passage that some indigenous cultures have required before a young man is acknowledged as an adult. Anthropologists describe these initiations as physical, psychological, and spiritual ordeals that are tests of courage and endurance. In such rites of passage, success is usual but not without risk to life, limb, and soul, which was also the case for Andy's surgery. The operation was successful, and the spirit in which my son made the passage was indeed admirable. Inspired by the title of Alice Walker's book of the same name, I thought of his surgical scars as "warrior marks."

Difficulties are soul-shaping; they can be lessons that lead us to know who we are, and they can stretch us into becoming larger souls and more authentic human beings than we were before. How we respond to unwanted and unchosen circumstances—such as those which lead to a medical diagnosis and need for surgery—may shape us as much as, or more than, the adversity itself.

We take up Psyche's journey as well as her lamp and knife once we face what is wrong and prepare ourselves for what we need to do. Like Psyche, once we are determined to know the truth and are prepared to act decisively, there is no turning back even when we are overwhelmed by difficulties and doubts. In the midst of an illness, treatment, or hospitalization that is a descent into the underworld, we may—like Psyche—find unexpected inner sources of courage, strength, and wisdom just when we need them. Qualities that are found, lessons that are taken to heart, shifts in attitude or changes that are made through surviving a life-threatening illness then reverberate through the whole of a person's life.

4

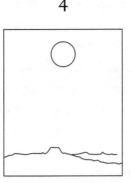

LIKE GREEN MEAT ON A HOOK

When Inanna went down through the seven gates into the Great Below, the proud and powerful goddess entered naked and bowed low, looked into the baleful eyes of death, and was struck down. Her body was hung on a hook to rot. She became a slab of green meat. This is a picture of how it feels to be reduced and humbled, powerless and without illusions, to be vulnerable and rejected, to feel putrid. There are phases of being ill in which people feel like Inanna on the hook, when the infected, dysfunctional, or malignant cellular level of their being permeates the soul, and they feel as if they were dead and rotting. This is what suffering can feel like to those who make a psychological descent to uncover sources of chronic depression and anxiety in the depth work I do as a Jungian analyst, as well.

This also powerfully parallels the experience that women and some men have had in abusive relationships that have stripped them of layers of self-esteem and psychological defense. There is physical, emotional, and spiritual battering in abusive relationships, and the most malignant of them can become life-threatening. The need to get away, the difficulty of doing so, and the effort to recover psychological health and not return have many similarities to what it takes to recover from a malignancy. To live with a chronic illness such as diabetes or hypertension when it gets out of control and escalates into life-threatening crises and repeated emergency room admissions, shares similarities—at the soul level—to the person who has repeated, increasingly serious, bouts with alcohol. To bottom out, one way or another, is a descent into suffering.

Anyone with a malignancy, a chronic illness, a drug or alcohol addiction, a mental illness, or trauma may identify with Inanna at this low point in the myth. You may have been depressed and anxious before you became ill. You may have been psychologically naked and bowed low before this, and the symptoms of the illness have further reduced your spirit. Sick physically, you may now feel as if the cells of your body were dying and rotting. And, the illness may do what psychological distress did not: it may cause you to go down into your own psychological depths, to be with the pain, wounding, and rage that is there—to that place in the psyche where a woman or a man is *both* suffering Inanna and suffering Ereshkigal.

Why did Inanna make this descent, anyway? What made her leave the Great Above where she was Queen of Heaven and Earth to descend into the underworld? When she knocked loudly at the gate to the Great Below and demanded that the door be opened for her, the gatekeeper asked, "Who are you?" and was told, "I am Inanna, Queen of Heaven, on my way to the East." When he asked, "Why has your heart led you on the road from which no traveler returns?" Inanna replied, "Because of my sister, Ereshkigal." Once she learned that her sister goddess Ereshkigal was suffering and in mourning, Inanna was compelled to make this descent, to be a witness.

Put in a medical context, Inanna's reason for unknowingly beginning a descent is like learning that something is physically wrong— "Ereshkigal is suffering" may translate into a suspicious finding on a routine physical examination, or noticing something oneself that cannot be ignored—and being compelled to go through the doors into the hospital, clinic, laboratory, or specialist's office to do whatever is required for the diagnosis and treatment.

Inanna's reason for making a descent is also metaphorically the same as why a person enters a psychotherapist's office: a need to know what lies below her usual level of consciousness, to find out what or which aspect of herself is suffering, to delve deeply into the grief and pain that lies in the Great Below. To knock at my office door in order to enter a depth psychological process is to knock at a gate to the underworld. Nightmares; repetitive dreams; unbidden thoughts, images, and impulses; pervasive anxiety; depression; inability to know what one really feels; deep unhappiness are some of the reasons for making a descent, through which it may be possible to be a witness, to feel, know, remember, and mourn what lies below. However compelling the psychological reasons are for making a descent, people often resist, using addictions to work, relationships, activity, television, alcohol, or other reality-distorting substances to avoid making a descent, as all of these are ways of keeping awareness of pain at bay. Unless psychological symptoms become so disabling that a person cannot function, it is possible to resist. Life-threatening illness, however, takes us out of ordinary life and into the underworld. A descent is then no longer an elective procedure.

Inanna described herself to the gatekeeper as being on her way to the East, which is a strange statement to make when she is seeking entry to the underworld; it makes symbolic sense, however. Dawn comes when the sun rises in the east, and hence the East represents rebirth, new life vulnerability, innocence, and hope. Descents into the underworld take a person into the realm of death, transformation, and rebirth. In a descent, there are symbolic deaths: death of some part of the old personality or former identity, the end of a particular hope or illusion. In a descent, something that has been buried in the psyche may be unearthed, remembered, and brought to life. There is a possibility of a spiritual or psychological resurrection.

Women who function well in the world of social and professional life resemble Inanna; they do well in the material world and are well connected to patriarchy, often as wives or daughters of traditional men. Ereshkigal, meanwhile, suffers in the underworld. Ereshkigal—as a contemporary archetype—represents inner or rejected or repressed aspects of an Inanna woman and of women in general. A woman who is more like Ereshkigal than Inanna has qualities and concerns that are introverted and unrelated, devalued and rejected; she is wounded and angry, often is depressed, can be ill, and is not allied with men with power. Ereshkigal is hidden in the underworld: socially invisible and discounted, manifested in public by the crazy or angry woman muttering to herself. Just as we avert our eyes from the street person who is being Ereshkigal, so do "nice women" avert their awareness from the Ereshkigal inside themselves; she is buried in the depressive mood, hidden in the physical symptom, or even in their good deeds that have shadowy origins. Nice women try to repress unacceptable hostile feelings, thoughts, and impulses; when they succeed in covering them up, unacceptable emotions and urges become hidden and out of conscious awareness; vague guilt remains, and the women often end up being extra nice to the very people toward whom they feel hostile.

"Nice women" learn to repress anger, especially on behalf of themselves, from an early age, when they are rejected and made to feel shame for having such feelings. As an aftermath, they wear mental blinders that keep them from noticing the demeaning of women in general or themselves in particular. Instead they themselves adopt these same negative attitudes. Thus nice women do not think well of women and do not consider them as worthy as men. For all the status they may have, such women suffer from low self-esteem, anxiety, and depression. This prejudicial attitude toward women and thus toward themselves comes as much from their mothers as from fathers and society. A mother with an inner sense of worthlessness passes it on to her daughters; the devaluation is passed down from one generation to the next.

The pain and rage of not being loved and valued for herself is excluded from consciousness, along with the feelings, talents, ambitions, and dreams that were not acceptable for her to have. Whatever was rejected and repressed in the psyche remains alive in the Great Below, in the symbolic figure of Ereshkigal, who suffers.

Ereshkigal harbors hatred toward Inanna, a metaphor for the self-hatred that lies below the surface of Inanna women who have been shaped by the need to do well in order to be acceptable. We all come into the world wanting to be loved, and when we are not, we settle for less: men usually for power and control over others; women for approval from others.

The Inanna-Ereshkigal configuration grows out of childhoods where performance, appearance, and social approval counted and were possible to achieve. Such women find ways to get approval—by the way they look, dress, are socially accepted and marry well, or by work, from good grades to professional success: approval comes from being Inanna. But their experiences (which is true for men as well) of being unloved, of being the recipient of parental neglect or abuse, of not being cherished for themselves, can be condensed into the symbolic figure of Ereshkigal. They look as good as Inanna on the surface, and keep their misery as Ereshkigal hidden in the underworld. Until they make a descent, Ereshkigal may be as hidden from themselves as from the world.

Illness makes it impossible to go on as Inanna. Going through the gates, stripped of all the accoutrements of Inanna, there is no longer any way to maintain the persona and the illusion and protection that position and accomplishments offered; naked, bowed low, feeling like a slab of green meat on a hook, a woman who can no longer be Inanna finds herself becoming Ereshkigal, and discovers the self-hatred, worthlessness, hostility, pain, and rage that she had avoided feeling and knowing, until now. Ereshkigal's fury lashes out at the situation. Rage, terror, and grief rise like waves and go through her. Rage moves from "I don't deserve this!" to "I brought it on myself!" There is rage at the unfairness, rage at oneself, and rage at others who go about their usual lives. There is terror about dying, fear of being in pain or potentially disfigured; and grief that their lives are irrevocably altered. Ereshkigal moans in pain. Once "nice women" feel their gorge rising, blinders drop away—they see how unconcerned or self-concerned others are, and they are angry. But anger and rage are uncomfortable feelings for them to have or express; these feelings are incompatible with being "nice." They also fear alienating people they are dependent upon, especially now that they are ill and afraid. Consequently, newfound anger is unpredictably expressed or suppressed: one moment, a woman is furious; the next occasion she stuffs it, or directs the anger against herself and becomes depressed and feels worthless. In the meantime, there are doctor's appointments, procedures, demands for decisions, life that has to go on, and the aftermath of coping with diagnosis and treatment. No longer able to be Inanna and being an angry, in-pain Ereshkigal, is the low point—in the lives of women with life-threatening illnesses as it is in the myth.

AIDS is a major initiation into the Inanna-Ereshkigal story. The initial diagnosis takes AIDS patients through the first gate. Each subsequent medical crisis, each new opportunistic disease is another gate, another stripping away of physical resistance, of psychological denial, further loss of health, more humbling; by the time there is physical disability from AIDS, Inanna's descent is all too familiar a story. Gay men with AIDS also know something about Ereshkigal; in a homophobic society, pain and rage at being rejected, feared, hated, and harassed goes with the territory, much of which is internalized. There is also more familiarity with inner female figures, and "queens" are part of the culture, which makes imagining and then accepting the truth of the myth easier for gay men than for men in general.

However, when it's possible to see with metaphoric eyes beyond the female figures of Inanna and Ereshkigal to what they represent, these two bear a striking resemblance to a psychological upperworld-underworld split in many traditional men.

When Inanna set off for the underworld, her loyal friend Ninshubur accompanied her to the first gate and received Inanna's instructions.

She was to wait there until Inanna returned, and if she did not return after three days and nights, Inanna's survival would depend on Ninshubur. Ninshubur, the third woman in the descent story, is described as Inanna's faithful servant, as her trustworthy and competent minister, warrior, messenger, general, and adviser. Ninshubur represents the third interior figure. As in the myth, Ninshubur needs to be active on behalf of a person who is in the midst of a descent into the underworld.

In spite of the emotional devastation and upheaval that a life-endangering diagnosis and treatment precipitates people into, there are decisions to be made and actions to be taken that require us also to function as Ninshubur while in the midst of descent. Ninshubur's loyalty is to her friend; competency and devotion are her characteristics. As an inner figure, Ninshubur needs to be a part of our character for us to be able to act on our own behalf; when *I* need to see the situation that *I* am in, and be able to act, seek help, and feel for *myself*, it is this Ninshubur quality that makes it possible. When a person is overwhelmed by the situation, or has never developed an inner Ninshubur, others can function as Ninshubur in helping us to see clearly and support us to do what we need to do. This can be done by a loyal friend or friends, a spouse, a therapist, or a support group.

When three days and three nights passed, and Inanna did not return—for she was now hanging on a hook in the underworld and had become a rotting piece of green meat—loyal Ninshubur followed her instructions exactly. Ninshubur was to lament her loudly, beat the drum in the assemblies so all would know, and seek help from the father gods. She appealed to each, saying, "Do not let your daughter Inanna be put to death in the underworld." The first two gods she approached could not be bothered with Inanna's plight and reacted in anger at even being asked for help. The third god was troubled and grieved, wanted to hear what had happened to Inanna, and immediately acted—in a curious way. He cleaned under his fingernails and brought forth the dirt and lint, or whatever was there, and fashioned two small creatures. They were neither male nor female and could fly through cracks in the seven gates unobserved, small enough not to be noticed, perhaps the size of flies. To one, he gave drops of the nectar of life; to the other, he gave crumbs of the food of life. He told them that they would find Ereshkigal moaning in pain, "with the cries of a woman about to give birth," unclothed, her breasts uncovered and her hair disheveled, and that they were to respond with compassion to her cries.

Each time Ereshkigal moaned in pain, "Oh! Oh! My inside!" they moaned, "Oh! Oh! Your inside!" Each time Ereshkigal moaned, "Oh! Oh! My outside!" they moaned, "Oh! Oh! Your outside!" When she cried out, "Oh! Oh! my belly!" and "Ohhhh! Oh! my back!" and "Ah! Ah! my heart!" and "Ahh! Ah! my breast!" they responded, empathically moaning, groaning, and sighing with her, and in doing so, they shared and witnessed her pain, until finally, her pain was gone, and she was also no longer the angry, death-bringing baleful goddess. Instead, she was now grateful and generous. She offered them a series of magnificent gifts—and to each, they responded with "We do not wish it," until she gave up and said, "Speak then! What do you wish?" And they answered that they would take "the corpse that hangs from the hook on the wall." Grateful Ereshkigal gave them the green, rotting corpse that was Inanna. One sprinkled drops of the water of life on the dead lips of Inanna, the other gave her crumbs of the food of life. Thus Inanna arose from the dead, ready to ascend from the Great Below and return to the Great Above.

If I were telling you this myth because you were in the midst of a descent, and you had really listened, it could serve as an initiation story, a metaphoric map for the journey that you know something about in the marrow of your bones. It is a story that can be taken to heart, long before the mind knows why. This was the case several years ago, when I told the story of Inanna and Ereshkigal to Helene Smith, Ph.D., the director of a cancer research center, who had in the previous few weeks been diagnosed with breast cancer and was just recovering from surgery when I saw her. Helene's research was on breast cancer, and this turn of events might have remained a bitter irony, a mockery that diminished the meaning of her lifework, had she not been able to see this illness as a rite of passage.

Helene told of her experience in "A Tale of Two Sisters" in a medical center publication.[1] She recounted that when she heard the story about Inanna's descent, "I cried for the first time and that was really the beginning of my healing."

She went on to say, "The meaning of the myth has taken me years to fully understand. I had a sister who died of cancer, and I had many difficulties with that relationship [this sister had been an Ereshkigal to Helene's Inanna, in the contrast between her life and Helene's professional and personal accomplishments and recognition in the world], so there was healing that was necessary for me to do at a symbolic level. But also, you see, we are all Ereshkigal."

Helene saw that the two sisters in the myth "are really the two sides of ourselves" that we need to bring together, make peace with, and show compassion for. "It's your negative side that will destroy your positive side unless you are willing to recognize yourself as having both. From there I started meditating, and bunches of flies (those compassionate creatures in the myth who empathized with suffering) came to me in meditation to bring me back from the underworld. It became a real healing for me."

The descent part of the Inanna myth—the going through the gates and giving up symbols of identity, persona, defenses; being stripped, humbled, struck down, and left hanging on a hook, feeling like so much dead meat—is the easy part of the story to understand as metaphor. In our suffering and losses, we have all been Inanna. It is much harder to accept that we are also Ereshkigal, because she is a combination of disowned, unacceptable, or undeveloped qualities that become known only through a descent, through which we give up illusions, stop denying the truth, and lose our former (often one-sided)

1. Susan Weiner with Helene Smith, "A Tale of Two Sisters" in *Ways of the Healer,* Fall 1994/Winter 1995 (San Francisco: Program of Medicine & Philosophy, California-Pacific Medical Center), pp. 8–10.

sense of ourselves. We may have projected these qualities upon others, or judged, rejected, scapegoated, and distanced ourselves from anyone who exemplified Ereshkigal.

Ereshkigal is wrathful, her baleful look can kill, and she can strike a death blow. She expresses raw emotions and pain. She is also a symbol of our fear of death and our fear of rejection. When we descend into our own underworld and find her in ourselves, our former image of ourselves and of reality has to die. Only through the ego-persona descent as Inanna and the encounter with the shadow that is Ereshkigal, can there be a possibility of symbolic resurrection or rebirth, which is the soul journey. There is a great risk that Ereshkigal in her raw pain and destructiveness will not just be known and felt temporarily, as part of the descent process, but that the patient with a life-threatening illness will become bitter, angry, isolated, rejecting, and alienated from her or his soul journey and from a common humanity that links us as well.

The small, androgynous creatures who flew through the gates like flies came to Ereshkigal, whose suffering gave her the appearance of a woman in the throes of labor; they saw and heard her pain and did not discount, minimize, question, or blame her. They expressed only compassion and stayed with her. In the presence of acceptance and compassion, Ereshkigal's pain and anger were transformed into gratitude, and as a result, Inanna could come back to life.

However, as the judges of the underworld informed her, "No one ascends from the underworld unmarked."

5

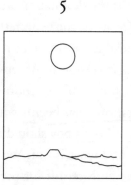

PROCRUSTEAN DISMEMBERMENT

Sometimes I wonder if a life-threatening illness or condition is a last-ditch opportunity to pay attention to soul needs for authentic expression, for creativity, for intimacy, for solitude, for retreat inward, for something significant to happen. Perhaps when all else has failed to call attention to pain at the soul level, disease not only may result but may become the means through which we go inward to find buried feelings and cut-off or dismembered aspects of ourselves.

There is a Greek story about Procrustes and his bed that I think of as a vivid metaphor about what happens to us, especially in the first half of our lives when establishing ourselves in the world of work and relationship are the developmental tasks. The procrustean bed is a short and simple myth. If you were traveling to Athens, you had to pass Procrustes and his bed. Procrustes would place you on his bed and see if you fit. Any part of you that did not fit, he cut off: whack! If you were too short for his bed, he would stretch you, as if on a medieval rack, until you did fit. In ancient times Athens was the center of commerce, art, politics, of civilization. Athens is a symbolic destination for anyone

63

on the road to success. It is the destination we are supposed to reach if we do well, the goal set for us by the expectations of others.

A particular family, social class, ethnic or religious group, or culture may have its own particular version of Athens, and it usually is different depending upon whether you were born male or female. It's the road of collective expectations that begins with assumptions of how a little girl should behave, of how a boy should act, about what is appropriate, what is accepted, and what is not. We are set on our particular road to Athens before we even set off for preschool: by then we have already been shaped by shame or fear of punishment; we have learned what gains approval and what provokes anger or rejection. School and schoolyard continue the process of adapting us to the standards of behavior and performance. We are shaped by our needs for acceptance and by our fears, and by the needs and fears of our parents, as well as by the standards of every group to which we aspire to belong. Every road to success or acceptability is a toll road with procrustean toll takers that separate us from parts and pieces of ourselves that do not fit. This may turn out to be a very high price to pay.

We take part in the dismemberment process when an aspect of ourselves is rejected by our family, and we, in turn, also reject it. Or when an attribute of our personality becomes associated with feelings of shame or humiliation, and is suppressed by us. Or when there is a threat of withdrawal of love, and we sacrifice a part of ourselves, so that we won't be abandoned. If we noticed things and asked innocent questions that provoked anger or voiced how we felt and were repeatedly told we did not feel this way, if we got into trouble for speaking the truth, or no one cared how we felt, then we may have been cut off or cut ourselves off from whole areas of perception and expression.

People learn to dissociate themselves from whatever it is about them that leads to pain and shame. How far underground this goes, whether awareness remains of what is hidden away, depends upon how conscious or unconscious we are. This procrustean process applies to memories that we decide we are better off forgetting. It applies to whole parts of ourselves that were not allowed to develop or even to what is not accepted now. Whatever we cut off is buried in the underworld, and like all contents of the psyche is still alive. When we make a descent into the underworld and find pieces and parts of ourselves that we abandoned or forgot, we are engaged in a process of re-membering that is about healing and wholeness.

Most conventionally successful people fit into the procrustean bed of family and cultural expectations, or stretched to fit in easily. Usually this means that accomplishing the tasks of the first half of adult life to do with social acceptance and competence goes smoothly. There is a susceptibility and thus a likelihood that the ego may become identified with the persona, with a role, or with work, and often the result is a one-sided person without much access to the inner world. To connect with others on something more than a persona level, one must know one's own depths, for it is soul that recognizes another soul. When a person has fit the procrustean bed all too well, the success at adaptation may get in the way of *individuation,* which is to have a personal, authentic individual life that grows out of the depths of who each of us is, what we value and love and know from within to be true.

Recovering Dismembered Parts of Ourselves

When a life-threatening illness is suspected or confirmed, the possibility arises that nothing will be the same again. Awareness comes that whatever was deferred while on the road to Athens, may never be lived. Promises made to oneself or to others may never be kept. Intentions carry no weight when there may be no future health or life. In waiting rooms, hospital rooms, and in long nights of interrupted sleep, memories and images arise, thoughts and feelings come. There may be regret, remorse, and anger at how one has lived or not lived. There is grief for people and passions that were cut out of one's life because they were inappropriate and shed along the way because they didn't conform to ambitions or were neglected and forgotten in the midst of personal and career moves. Or perhaps they'd been sacrificed to keep the peace, to avert the jealousy, envy, fear, or resentment of a spouse or parent.

A life-threatening illness can expose the dismembered parts of ourselves that were cut off and buried in the unconscious. For many women, especially those who have been depressed, anxious, or addicted to activity, alcohol, or anything that has kept them from feeling, the encounter with Ereshkigal is potentially transformative. Ereshkigal was not nice or hospitable. She was in pain. She was angry, and she could strike someone dead—characteristics and feelings that many nice women and good-natured men repress and keep hidden from themselves and others. When her suffering was witnessed, and she was heard and responded to with compassion, it changed her. She became grateful and generous, and could bestow important gifts. Ereshkigal is powerful. Integrating her strengths empowers a person to be decisive, to mete out rewards and punishments.

Integrating Ereshkigal

A woman who meets her interior Ereshkigal and integrates feelings and power that were repressed and buried, emerges from the underworld, as did Inanna, changed. Brought back to life, a resurrected Inanna ascended to the upperworld with demons clinging to her, ready to leap off and claim whomever she designated to return with them to the underworld in her place.

The first person they met was loyal Ninshubur, wearing sackcloth. The demons said, "Walk on, Inanna, we will take Ninshubur in your place." Inanna responded, "No! Ninshubur is my constant support." First she described Ninshubur's wisdom and her warrior qualities. Then she enumerated what Ninshubur had done on her behalf, and finally she said to the demons, "Because of her, my life was saved. I will never give Ninshubur to you."

Inanna and the demons then were met by her son Shara, and next by her son Lulal. Both were dressed in sackcloth, in mourning for Inanna. The demons were ready to take first one and then the other. Inanna told the demons who they were to her, and would not give them up. Finally, Inanna and the demons entered her city, and there she saw her husband, Dumazi, dressed in his magnificent garments and sitting on the throne (obviously not in mourning for Inanna). "Inanna fastened on Dumazi the eye of death. She spoke against him the word of wrath. She uttered against him the cry of guilt: Take him! Take Dumazi away!"

Anyone who has had an encounter with the possibility of death has all her significant relationships tested. Who suffers with her? Who is really affected by the possibility that she may not return from a descent, that she may not survive the ordeal and be returned to health? Friend, family member, spouse? To whom does she really matter? With the ability to discern how others feel about her and to know what others mean to her, Inanna acts. She wields the power she has gained in the underworld: she can feel wrath and unleash demons and choose who shall be banished from her life and who shall be kept in it.

The Exceptional Patient

Translated from myth into life, a life-threatening illness may be the means through which discernment and wrath become conscious. When qualities symbolized by Ereshkigal are no long dismembered, when feelings and perceptions are no longer cut off from awareness and are instead acknowledged and expressed, a transformation has taken place. No longer is anger repressed and turned into depression, nor is painful reality buried under addictions that numb feelings. The net result is *a person who expresses emotions and can act on his or her own behalf.*

These are characteristics needed to become "exceptional patients" that Dr. Bernie Siegel described in *Love, Medicine and Miracles*, those people with life-threatening illnesses who are most likely to get well. These are also the patients whom physicians usually consider difficult or uncooperative because they ask questions, express their emotions, and become specialists in their own care.[1]

1. Bernie S. Siegel, *Love, Medicine and Miracles: Lessons Learned About Self-Healing from a Surgeon's Experience with Exceptional Patients* (New York: Harper & Row, 1986), pp. 23–25.

Siegel described three types of patients. He characterized about 15 or 20 percent as unconsciously or consciously wishing to die. These were people who on some level welcomed cancer or another serious illness as a way out of their problems. They show no signs of stress when they find out their diagnosis. As the doctor is struggling to get them well, they are resisting and trying to die. If you ask them how they are, they say, "Fine." Or what is troubling them? "Nothing."

The majority fit into the middle of the spectrum of patients, about 60 to 70 percent. Siegel characterizes them as performing to satisfy the physician. This group does what they're told—unless the doctor suggests radical changes in their lifestyle. It never occurs to them to question the doctor's decisions or strike out on their own.

At the other extreme are the 15 to 20 percent who are exceptional. They want to know every detail of their X-ray reports, the meaning of every number in their lab test printouts, what their treatment options are, why a particular choice is recommended, and what the side effects may be. They seek second opinions and look into the alternatives. They put themselves into the process of getting well; whatever they believe will help them get well that they can do, they will. They can be found in support groups, meditating, visualizing, delving into psychotherapies, expressing what they feel, changing their lifestyles and what they eat. They are activists on their own behalf who act on the belief that they can make a difference in the outcome of their disease, and they do.

Siegel reviewed research that supported this. In one study of thirty-five women with metastatic breast cancer, the long-term survivors had poor relationships with their physicians as judged by the physicians; they asked a lot of questions and expressed their emotions. In another study, aggressive "bad" patients tended to have more killer T cells, the white cells that seek and destroy cancer cells, than did docile "good" patients. In a third report, there was a ten-year survival rate of 75 percent among cancer patients who reacted to the diagnosis with a fighting spirit, compared with a 22 percent survival rate among those who responded with stoic acceptance or feelings of helplessness or hopelessness.

Gratitude and Wholeness

Recovery of parts of ourselves that were repressed when they were not welcomed by others, has to do with becoming a whole person with a range and depth of feelings, the ability to discern and choose, to express feelings and act on them. We come to trust what we know to be true or right for ourselves as a result.

A life-threatening illness can lead to a major change in direction. It can result in charting a personal course instead of proceeding on that road to Athens with its collective procrustean standards. When she did not die at age thirty-five, a woman physician I interned with at Los Angeles General Hospital considered every year thereafter a gift of life. Up to then, she had spent most of her adult life overworking as a medical student, intern, and resident, and then as a radiologist. She had spent more time in hospitals than anywhere else, had paid scant attention to developing other interests or talents, and had never married. Now, she took time for herself.

Whenever possible, she opted for time rather than money, and with partners in her professional corporation willing to make the trade, she spent every summer in Maine working with clay, sculpting, and making what she wanted on the potter's wheel. She was doing what she loved, creating and centering herself as well as the clay, instead of being professionally ambitious. She traveled widely, mindful that this opportunity was part of the gift of time that still remained. And she cultivated an inner life that was shaped by her awareness and familiarity with death. She had over fifteen good years before she died.

People who have made a descent as she did, and consequently know the value of the inner world and the nearness of the otherworld, incorporate what they know into conscious life. Soul is a presence in them, and somehow others feel the authenticity that accompanies soul. Even in the last months of her life, friends who visited thinking she might need cheering up, immediately found that not only was this not the case, but there was solace for them in her company. She approached death with serenity.

Life-Threatening Illness as a Soul-Shaping Experience

When life is lived superficially or is almost entirely outer-directed, something has to happen that leads to soul-searching. Until then, there may be very little communication between the upperworld and underworld, between the inner world of the personal and collective unconscious and the outer-world concerns of the ego. Layers of facade, of entitlement, and privilege that were built up over the years have no bearing on the occurrence or progression of an illness, and do not adequately prepare a person for the underworld descent—stripped like Inanna of the accoutrements of position or power. Years of taking care of the needs of others, or of devotion to work or to a cause, during which there has been virtually no attention paid to inner life or spiritual life, come to an end with a life-threatening illness, plunging a person into inactivity and into the underworld.

Illness raises questions: *Who are you when you stop doing?* When you cannot be productive or are no longer indispensable to others? When you can no longer go on as before because you are sick, when you lose status? Who are you when you can't be a caretaker or a boss or do your job, whatever that might be? Do *you* matter?

Illness takes us out of our minds and into our bodies. The upperworld that we leave is also the mental clarity of our former selves. Pain and medications, depression and fear, the side effects of having a life-threatening illness and being treated for it affects memory, the attention to details, the capacity to think well, to focus our minds and care about intellectual pursuits. Illnesses are mind-threatening as well as life-threatening. Even the most mundane transient illnesses muddle the mind; a cold or a touch of the flu forces us to attend to our bodies and shift our focus.

I think that these very impairments of mind and body may turn out to be the means through which it becomes possible to make changes in life that liberate us from soul-consuming relationships and work. I suspect that being adrift mentally and unable to work as usual plays a significant part in healing the soul. Illness takes us into a spiritual realm, where prayer belongs, and much of our waking hours have a meditative or dreamy quality. As spiritual beings on a human path, we yearn for connection with our own divine nature, and it is forgetting this that makes us susceptible to addictions, including the need always to be doing something, no matter how empty the activity.

Longings to be taken care of or close to others, which we might otherwise deny, also come to the surface when we are sick. People are vulnerable and need others, but this human reality is denied by many driven people—especially men, but increasingly by women as well—who are on the run from this dependent facet of themselves. I mused upon this at a memorial service for a man who had died of AIDS. Prior to his illness he successfully kept people at a distance with his brilliance and arrogance, but in the years just before his death he took down the wall that separated him from others, as well as the wall within himself that had kept his loving, trusting nature in the closet, hidden from expression. Before, he had been intimidating; revealing this part of himself, he became beloved.

Remembering our own nature may come through inner work done with a psychological or spiritual counselor, in meditation, in therapy, or as I increasingly see happening, in circles of people who are open to each other and to an invisible presence or spiritual energy. It is this energy that makes the circle a trustworthy container, a *temenos* or sanctuary, where it is safe to tell the truth of what you feel or perceive or have done. Spirit enters relationship between and among people, when we drop below the level of the ego/persona, and relate directly to the Self within: "where two or more are gathered in my name, there I shall be also" is a biblical promise and an archetypal reality.

Healing Circles

At a recent retreat, I sat in a circle of twenty-seven women, twenty of whom were surviving cancer, and all of whom were in a major transition time in their lives. The future was uncertain (as it actually is for everyone, but individuals in this group really knew it). They spoke of what they had been through and still were in the midst of, what their lives had been before the cancer, and the changes they had made since. I heard variations of two stories from the majority of them. The first and clearest about themselves were self-identified workaholics. They spoke of how work had been consuming, not just because of the sixty or eighty hours spent doing work each week, but because work had been the center of their lives. The second common story was of being consumed by caring for others. In the period that led to the diagnosis, these women had been taking care of a sick parent, an ailing husband, or living with an alcoholic, often while also being a provider. I had the impression that work or relationships that began by being important to them had gradually taken them over, until they couldn't quit and they couldn't go on and on and on, either. Cancer had made it impossible to continue making either work or another person's needs the center of their lives. It required that they look after themselves and be more dependent on others than they ever had been.

Each woman in the circle was a unique individual, and yet as we sat together I could say that every woman also represented a facet of each of us, and by speaking, voiced something for someone else as well as for herself. We met at a soul level and told the truth of how we felt and knew from experience. It was raining and quite dreary, as it had been for weeks, and one of the founders of the sponsoring organization had died of metastatic breast cancer just two days before our meeting, and another had recently discovered a new lump. Still, there was a spiritual glow and an emotional warmth; it was as if Hestia, the Goddess of the Hearth and Temple, was present in the candle flame in the middle of our circle. There was laughter and tears and soul. The circle was an alchemical vessel for soul growth, it was a nurturing and comforting container within which there was more than enough good mother to go around. We had left the ordinary world to come together, and it felt as if there was a heartful luminosity that touched us and came from us, *and* we were in the underworld or otherworld, re-membering human experiences of being around the warmth and safety of a fire, sheltered from the elements outside.

Couples who together face a life-threatening illness that one of them has, and make a descent together, describe how they unexpectedly find themselves in a magic circle of trust and love in the midst of an underworld experience, as well. Nothing is taken for granted, feelings are put into words, and with each new crisis, a new commitment to be there emotionally and vulnerably for the other is made by each of them. When there is no protective holding back, the soul-to-soul connection that grows is beautiful and tender. Friends and family members enter this alchemical vessel as well when they are open-souled, in an I-Thou relationship where each feels the other is beloved. In a time of descent, a depth of connection occurs that might otherwise not have developed or not have been expressed.

The giving and receiving of unconditional love, of knowing in that moment that we are truly loved just as we are, and able to love with our whole heart in return, is a human epiphany imbued by grace. From the perspective of the soul, when we love unconditionally, we are a channel for grace. Grace is that ineffable mysterious healing presence or energy that makes moments sacramental or holy, full of soul.

Experiencing Unconditional Love

I think about an intimation of this that I felt in Calcutta at Mother Teresa's Hospice for the Destitute and Dying. Outside the streets were teeming with people on foot, on bicycles, in honking vehicles; there were stalls and street hawkers, and the temple of Kali close by. My senses felt assaulted by the cacophony, by the smells and the heat, by the heavy brown air that hung over the city, and by the visual juxtaposition of it all. Passing into the hospice, through the doors and thick walls, was like entering another world of quiet and serenity, a cool and calm temple. It was laid out like the old general hospital open wards, one for men, another for women. Several sisters in saris were ministering to the needs of people who were lying on pallets close to the floor. A volunteer whom I recognized as Jerry Brown, the former governor of California, was washing a man who had recently been brought in. Never, in any hospital setting, had I ever felt such peace. Here were people who had been picked up on the sidewalks, gutters, or streets of Calcutta, near dead. Every day, a vehicle made the rounds bringing such people to the hospice. While many did die there, others eventually became well enough to leave.

They had been brought to the hospice so that once before they died, they could experience total and unconditional love, not through someone who knew them personally, but through the heart, soul, touch, and eyes of these sisters and volunteers, who saw the beauty of their souls, even despite the wretched condition of their bodies and often their lives. They were lying on their pallets, and in the very air of serenity, they breathed in something ineffable and soul comforting. I wonder, might this be a glimpse of what we come to experience in this human life? Unconditional love that warms the heart and soul, love that is divine and yet humanly given and received? A deep peace that comes from being held in invisible arms, a feeling of being beloved that is initiated by loving human touch? At the threshold of death, to trust and not be fearful?

I have mused upon the notion that all spiritual practices have to do with the recovery of innocence and how a life-threatening illness may lead to this, and I wonder if it is this recovery of innocence that accounts for the deep serenity at Mother Teresa's hospice. Might these men and women, so lovingly bathed and cared for, now resting in a fetal position on their pallets, who within a day or so may die in peace, be sleeping the sleep of the innocent?

The poorest of the poor who were picked up destitute and dying on the streets of Calcutta, to lie at peace on a pallet, have an essentially similar experience to women in healing circles, or cancer patients who go to healing communities such as Commonweal or the Center for

Attitudinal Change, or AIDS patients who live in residential hospices. They partake of unconditional love, and feel acceptable and whole. Healing a fragmented soul results.

Procrustean expectations and standards, in contrast, make it impossible for us to feel both acceptable *and* whole. In a circle of unconditional love, it becomes possible to retrieve what we and others rejected of ourselves. I believe that it includes an innocence we came into the world with, anticipating we would be loved.

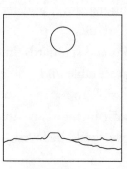

6

ILLNESS AS A TURNING POINT

time-out is called by teams when they are behind, and there is a need to stop the clock, pause for breath, consider a new strategy, or bring in a new player. We wonder, as they huddle, if they can possibly come from behind to win. The patients Lawrence LeShan described in *Cancer as a Turning Point* were in an analogous situation. Their poor prognoses meant the clock was running out. At this juncture, they began doing psychotherapy work with LeShan.

LeShan asked them soul-searching questions, ones that cannot be answered by the intellect, but require delving deeply and returning with forgotten memories of joy and contentment, and being truthful about the numbing despair or lack of meaning (which are related) in their lives. Life lacks a juicy quality when such is so. In his thirty-five years of working with cancer patients, LeShan, a research and clinical psychologist, found how psychological change along with medical treatment mobilizes a compromised immune system for healing. He found that enhancing life extends life.

He asked: *What kind of life and lifestyle would make you glad to get up in the morning and go to bed at night "good tired"? What would give you the maximum zest and enthusiasm in life? What kind of life can you conceive of that would use all of you, would be harmonious with you physically, psychologically, and spiritually? What kind of life would be "natural" for your entire being? How would you live if you could adjust the world to yourself?*[1]

Finding Your Myth

LeShan's questions reminded me of Joseph Campbell's response to a young man in an audience who had listened to him speak about the necessity of finding your own myth. For, finding your own myth and finding answers to LeShan's questions are variations on the same theme: discover who you are and live according to that truth.

The man asked Campbell, "How is a person to go about finding his or her myth?"

Campbell responded with a question of his own: "Where is your deepest sense of harmony and bliss?"

"I don't know—I'm not sure" was the reply.

"Find it," Campbell sang back, "and then follow it."[2]

Campbell was often quoted and sometimes criticized for saying, "Follow your bliss," by people who did not understand what it might mean to do so. Far from irresponsibly moving from one hedonistic pleasure to another, it was advice ideally leading to a lifetime's commitment—as it did for Campbell when he followed his love of mythology.

The answers to LeShan's questions and Campbell's answer to the young man come from what gives you *your deepest sense of harmony and bliss,* which has to do with soul. Psychologically, there is harmony and

1. All references to LeShan's work are taken from Lawrence LeShan, *Cancer as a Turning Point: A Handbook for People with Cancer, Their Families, and Health Professionals,* rev. ed. (New York: Plume, 1994).
2. Keith Thompson, "Myths as Souls of the World," review of *Inner Reaches of Outer Space,* by Joseph Campbell, *Noetics Sciences Review* (Winter 1986), p. 24.

bliss when what you are doing and being is a personal expression of an archetypal pattern through which the Self is felt. You feel centered, you have a sense of being *yourself,* there are moments that are sacred, and there is meaning in your life.

Archetypes

C. G. Jung introduced the concept of archetypes into psychology. They are innate predispositions that affect personality, relationships, and work. When life feels stale and meaningless, and something seems fundamentally wrong about how you are living and what you are doing, there are likely discrepancies between the archetypes in you and the visible roles, discrepancies between the surface layer and what you feel and are inside. I was drawn to the Greek gods and goddesses as a means of describing these inner patterns, and did so in *Goddesses in Everywoman* and *Gods in Everyman.* Living an authentic life, finding meaning, and having a personal myth are all connected with this archetypal layer of the psyche. Personal answers to LeShan's questions are found when you discover these archetypal sources of meaning. But you don't have to know the names of your archetypes or have a title for your myth: your truth is your myth. It's where *you* find harmony and bliss.

Harmony is being on the right path, being one with it—making a living doing work that is absorbing and consistent with your personal values, doing what you have a gift for. Harmony is being with a partner or companions or alone, with animals or with nature, in a particular city or country or place, and having a sense of "ringing true" there. Harmony is experiencing deep grief that corresponds to deep loss. Harmony is uninhibited, unself-conscious spontaneity, the immediacy of laughter, the welling up of tears. Harmony happens when behavior and belief come together, when inner archetypal life and outer life are expressions of each other, and we are being true to who we are. And only we can know: "I feel at home here," "I am totally absorbed doing this," "It gives me joy," "I love you," "This is bliss."

Bliss and joy come in moments of living our highest truth—moments when what we do is consistent with our archetypal depths. It's when we are most authentic and trusting, and feel that whatever we are doing, which can be quite ordinary, is nonetheless sacred. This is when we sense that we are part of something divine that is in us and is everywhere.

Innate Aptitudes

Each of us is born with innate talents and aptitudes that go unrecognized and undeveloped until and unless there are opportunities for expression. Classrooms and schoolyards, families and workplaces reward and recognize only some abilities. There are many kinds of intelligence and different ways of perceiving, and yet only some are encouraged. There are many kinds of talents, and only some are valued. School boards decided what we could learn, how it would be taught, and when it would appear in the curriculum. Parents decided what lessons we should take after school. If we were lucky, maybe something we were supposed to learn dovetailed with what we had a talent for, and we loved and probably excelled at it.

Work (as well as life) that calls upon us to use and develop our innate gifts is personally meaningful. Work that interests us, challenges us to grow, and provides opportunities for us to be creative engages us in life. We feel authentic and true to ourselves when we do such work. When what we do is what we love, work is an expression of our true nature.

Recovery from life-threatening illnesses may depend upon finding what our aptitudes are. Here, the kind of aptitude testing that lets us explore a range of possibilities in order to uncover natural aptitudes, discover how our particular mind works, and reflect back to us what we innately prefer can point the way.

Would it, for example, be fun or frustrating for you to watch someone fold a sheet of paper, stick a pencil through the layers, and then be asked to point to the particular drawing among several that shows where the holes would be in the paper, if it were now unfolded and flat?[3] This is a test about spatial aptitude that is a delightful game for those with such a gift.

3. This test was given by the Johnson O'Conner Research Foundation, Inc.

Fun or frustrating are two contrasting *subjective* adjectives. It's fun to speculate or stretch an aspect of your mind, or to try a physical task that requires dexterity, or match colors or sounds, or pairs of words that mean something—if these tasks call up abilities that you have. It's very frustrating to not be able to excel, even if you try and practice, because this is just not one of your particular talents. It's hard to not have effort pay off in personal satisfaction. It's no fun to be a square peg in a round hole, even if you can do what is called for well enough to pass.

LeShan's patients went into long-term remissions by finding a zest for life that in turn affected the healing response of the body. An enthusiasm for life was an essential element: in my understanding, this happens when the soul becomes engaged in life and life has a purpose. *Enthusiasm* for life comes when we become infused by spirit or divinity; the word is derived from *en-theos* (Greek for "god"). I don't think it's possible to be genuinely enthusiastic unless we are also being authentically ourselves. This is when we are true to our particular aptitudes and archetypes.

Inner Sources of a Creative Life

LeShan characterized those individuals for whom cancer was a turning point as suffering from "foiled creative fire." By finding answers and making changes toward lives that went farther in expressing their own authentic selves, their creativity, enthusiasm, and vitality were rekindled. Approximately half of them, seen by him over a period of thirty years, went into long-term remissions and were alive when he wrote of his work with them.

For many of us, finding personal answers to LeShan's questions is made difficult by an ingrained habit of putting others' needs before our own or having self-esteem be synonymous with productivity, or discounting ourselves because others did so, and, in general, making small and large, often shame-based procrustean-bed decisions that cut us off from what really matters to us.

Sources of pleasure which lie dismembered, forgotten, and buried in the underworld have to be recovered. Seeds of creativity, uncultivated talents, forgotten yearnings, aborted dreams, and wisdom can be found there. On making a descent, the riches we find there are parts and pieces of our dismembered selves, the human inheritance of the symbolic and archetypal realm of the collective unconscious.

In the dim light of the underworld, the ego and intellect are of little use. This is the realm of soul, and it is the heart that aids us in finding gold in this dark place—once we shed the leaden weight of an inauthentic life. Paradoxically, once we acknowledge how alienated we are from living a meaningful life, how cut off we feel from our own depths, how little we love, how barren and empty our lives are, we begin to penetrate the darkness and find stirrings of heartfelt movement. Physical or emotional dysfunction and disease can be a gateway into the underworld, where pain *and* love have been hidden.

Preceding the appearance of physical and psychological disease, there has often been a period of months or years that resembles winter in northern climates. Winter is a time when nothing grows, when there is no creativity and nothing young and vulnerable comes to the surface, when life is not green and juicy. It is the psychological equivalent of a wasteland, a time of grayness, of feeling trapped in a static life. While pain and anger and grief may be buried below the surface and need to be unearthed, spring may never come if what ails the person is a life-threatening physical illness and the focus of psychotherapy is on negative childhood experiences and pathological motivations.

Working with traditional Freudian, psychoanalytical therapy methods and concepts, LeShan found that "none of my patients was getting better! They might look forward to my visits, they might even feel better afterward, but they kept right on dying at the same rate as if I were not involved with them at all." LeShan has concluded that any psychotherapy process (not just Freudian) that focuses on "What's wrong with this patient? How did he or she get this way? and What can be done about it?" which can be effective for a wide variety of emotional or cognitive problems, is not effective with cancer patients. *"It simply does not mobilize the person's self-healing abilities and bring them to the aid of the medical program."*

What Is True for You?

The therapeutic approach that LeShan developed in his research with cancer patients is based on entirely different questions. These are:

> What is right with this person? What are his (or her) special and unique ways of being, relating, creating, that are his own and natural ways to live? What is his special music to beat out in life, his unique song to sing so that when he is singing it he is glad to get up in the morning and glad to go to bed at night? What style of life would give him zest, enthusiasm, involvement?
>
> How can we work together to find these ways of being, relating, and creating? What has blocked their perception and/or expression in the past? How can we work together so that the person moves more and more in this direction until he is living such a full and zestful life that he has no more time or energy for psychotherapy?

While LeShan begins his inquiry with "What's right with this person?" instead of "What's wrong with this person?" his further questions all have to do with being special and being unique, not with a rightness or wrongness at all. *"What is true for this person?"* is, I believe, at the heart of his work, and of all psychological and spiritual work to do with individuation. It is at the heart of the depth psychological work that I have been doing—or learning to do with individuals—over the past thirty years. It is an undoing of the medical, psychiatric, and psychoanalytic perspective that concerns itself with making a pathological diagnosis, and instead focuses on resurrecting the thwarted sense of meaning and purpose that underlies the psychological or physical disease.

Might each life have a purpose? And might the uniqueness of the circumstances of our particular life, with its suffering, and our particular talents and loves, with its satisfactions and joy, be a key to what gives us a sense of purpose and path? And once we find what is true for us and live it, might this extend life?

I think LeShan's work points to this. I think the psychotherapy that leads cancer patients who might otherwise have died into a long-term remission begins with love as an essential ingredient in the process. Seek a therapist who loves the work, whose soul and heart are in it. Someone who can see beauty, vulnerability, and courage and care for these qualities. Someone for whom psychotherapy is his or her own soul work. For how can a therapist help someone else find soul in life, if that therapist has not found it himself or herself? When your life depends upon finding meaning, creativity, joy in life, the guide to your process has to have found his or her own way there.

When Michelangelo looked at a block of raw marble, he could see a figure imprisoned within it. With his talent and the tools of a sculptor, he brought forth the beauty, power, and magnificence of the figure that he saw and made it visible to all of us. A psychotherapist needs to have a similar eye to help free what is true in a person. For there to be an alchemy in the work of therapist or sculptor, there must not only be training and experience but also an ability to see potential and beauty. I believe that the soul, not the mind, recognizes these qualities.

Human warmth and emotion, compassion for us from another and for ourselves, brings spring thaws to winter wastelands. Denial and resistance to the truth begin to crack like ice that is thinning, to free the life that we felt we had to bury. Lying below frozen soil, covered by winter snow, lie dormant roots, bulbs, and seeds in need of rain and sun, which are like the potential blossoming of life-affirming possibilities, buried and forgotten in the psyche. It is love that reconnects us to soul, soul work, soul kin; it is love of what we are doing and love of who we are with that gives us a sense of having a place in the universe, of belonging. Love leads us toward what gives us bliss and harmony, purpose and meaning, and this can have a positive effect on medical conditions that might otherwise be fatal.

Achieving Detente Between Disease and Health

There are many illnesses that are potentially fatal, not just cancer. Other diseases can also progress and become terminal. Hypertension, diabetes, and autoimmune diseases do not metastasize, but they affect the entire body and can cause an organ to fail. Many diseases and infections spread, if they are unchecked, until they are fatal. Numerous other illnesses besides many cancers and AIDS are not curable, but are kept under control, their effects staved off for years and years. This is so for major psychiatric illnesses as well. Such patients stay in good or at least fair health if they attend consciously to what keeps them healthy *and* are lucky.

The collective mind-set or attitude toward a disease has a great deal to do with the psychological impact of a particular diagnosis. Expectations are powerful. The word *cancer* has a frightening effect on most people, far more than the names of any of the other chronic, often progressive diseases (except AIDS), that may, for a particular individual, be quite fatal.

The collective mind-set about cancers that have spread beyond the original site, especially when they have gone into bones or to other organs, often resembles that of a voodoo-believing community on hearing that someone has been hexed. One woman whose breast cancer had gone into her bones described a conversation with a young mother that was interrupted by her small son. On hearing who his mother was talking to on the phone, the little boy piped up, loud enough to be heard on the other end, "Isn't she dead yet?" Obviously, this child was repeating behind-the-back talk that reflected the assumption that metastatic cancer is as much a sudden death sentence as a hex is in a voodoo-believing community.

Exceptional patients such as the ones Dr. Siegel described do not accept collective or conventional assumptions and are willing to make major changes in their lives to stay alive and healthy, and exceptional psychotherapists such as Dr. LeShan help their clients to do so. The turning point begins with the belief that it is possible and taking action to bring this about.

Medicine is able to do a great deal, often dramatically, yet the return of health depends upon a great many other factors after medical intervention. Physical health improves when emotional outlook improves, when there are spiritual resources, good nutrition, and exercise, when noxious influences are removed, when people have something to live for, and when they do what will help them to be healthy.

A good example is Dr. Dean Ornish's approach to treating heart disease.[4] By following a vegetarian diet with a very low fat intake, exercising regularly, doing yoga and meditation, and having group support, it is possible to avoid surgery and reverse heart disease. Ornish's patients have actually reversed the disease process: blockages in arteries have decreased in size, and blood flow has improved. It has worked for people who were so sick that they couldn't walk across a room without experiencing chest pain.

LeShan's patients with long-term remissions and others are living rebuttals to the usual mind-set about metastatic cancer. They must be able to do so because the cancer and the body's defenses arrive at some sort of detente, like a political balance of power. Progression of disease stops when the forces of health can resist the forces of disease. With most medical and psychiatric disease, the same principle applies. Whether the metaphor is about balancing scales, or a tug-of-war, or a battlefield, or political detente, or putting out a fire, recovery depends upon the body and soul's ability to resist and then tip the balance toward health.

The turning point toward health for many individuals who have diseases that are demoralizing and depleting happens at the soul level. It has to do with discovering reasons to live, a will that is determined to do so, faith that it is possible, and wise choices about what to do. People are looking in all the wrong places for reasons to live when they look outward and seek to know with their intellect. The heart needs to be

4. Dean Ornish, M.D., *Dr. Dean Ornish's Program for Reversing Heart Disease: The Only System Scientifically Proven to Reverse Heart Disease Without Drugs or Surgery* (New York: Ballantine, 1990).

consulted. The beginning place to look in the search for meaning is inward.

How do we know what matters to us? How do we know what would make us glad to get up in the morning, absorb us, and allow us to go to bed "good" tired. How do we know what we love—when we have spent years not listening to the protestations of our bodies, our feelings, or our dreams, or ignoring inner messages of deep unhappiness?

Of all the ways that we might know, I have come to trust most the characteristics of time as a measure or indicator.

Kairos *and* Kronos

When love is actively present, we are absorbed in what we are doing and who we are with. Time takes on a different quality, and we often lose track of it. Recall when you were in love, how time passed: hours could seem like minutes, minutes could seem like hours, time could stand still. Whenever we are engaged in something that is soul-satisfying or of the heart, this is so.

The Greeks had two words for time: *kairos* and *kronos*. When we participate in time and therefore lose our sense of time passing, we are in *kairos;* here we are totally absorbed and in the present moment, which may actually stretch out over hours. Whenever we are in love with what we are doing or who we are with, whenever we are totally absorbed, engaged, and fascinated, we are in *kairos*. Creativity that taps into the depths allowing the person to be the soul through whom the words or music or answers come, happens in *kairos,* as does listening to words or music which seem to be expressions of ourselves: it is ". . . *music heard so deeply that it is not heard at all, but you are the music while the music lasts.*"[5]

Kairos is soul-nourishing time. Whatever we do in *kairos* is soul-satisfying *for us*. When I pull weeds and plant flowers in the spring, nothing else exists except the earth under my knees, and nothing else is on

5. T. S. Eliot, "The Dry Salvages," in *Four Quartets* (New York: Harcourt Brace Jovanovich, 1943, 1971), p. 44.

my mind; snorkeling in warm and safe Caribbean waters, I am like a fish myself, effortlessly following my eyes that see this beautiful fish or that coral formation or those translucent little fishes swimming in a school. Sometimes, just making a stew on a cold, foggy day brings me into *kairos*. Almost everyone has something equivalent. As I think of the people I know, it's needlepoint for one, sewing for another, chopping firewood, fly fishing, tinkering under a hood, playing the bass guitar, sketching, even cleaning house. Something that is onerous, difficult, or boring for one person is bliss and harmony for another.

What takes you into *kairos*? When do you lose track of time? What is it that nourishes your soul?

In the judgment of others (within ourselves and outside), to be absorbed in such unproductive activities is a waste of valuable time, rather than rich in and of itself. The practice of clearing one's mind is a goal of meditation, it is the essence of any soul-nourishing activity. It is *"a condition of complete simplicity (costing not less than everything)"*[6] when we do so. In *kairos*, there is only the present moment. In order to have it, we have to let go of everything else.

The second designation for time, *kronos*, refers to measured time. It's what we usually mean when we think about time. It's calendar time, clock time, deadlines; it's time we keep track of, and make appointments in; it's the Week-at-a-Glance book we are lost without; it's what we don't ever seem to have enough of to get everything that needs to be done, done. It's what oppressed you in classrooms when you wanted the class to end, or the semester to be over. We get the word *chronometer,* another name for a clock, from *chronos;* named also after Chronos or Kronos, the Greek god who swallowed his children as soon as they were born. *Kronos* is symbolized by the newborn baby that comes in on January 1 of each new year, and goes out a bent over old man with a beard on December 31; Father Time. *Chronos* is linear time, what we bill others for, equated often with money as in "time is money."

When you work for a paycheck and do not do work you love, when

6. Eliot, *Four Quartets*, p. 59.

you are dutifully making an appearance and wish you were somewhere else, when you seem to be "putting in time," rather than living, daily life is a burden. In contrast, when you are doing work that absorbs you body and soul, work that uses your talents and matters to you, then no matter how difficult or demanding it is, your work will have a quality of creative play to it, and there are moments of pure gold, when you make a discovery that clicks for you and have the joy in the doing of it. To find such work is one of the answers to the question: "What kind of life would make you glad to get up in the morning?"

Only you—no one else—can answer this question or any of the others that LeShan poses. To grasp the notion of *kairos* versus *kronos* is a starting place, a way of identifying through your own experiences what is soulful. In the midst of simple, satisfying, creative, or contemplative tasks that are soul-nourishing, you may find yourself remembering more of what you once loved, and being led by memory to further sources of meaning.

The very experience of *kairos* has an effect in everyday life of centering us, which in turn makes us feel as if we are in harmony with ourselves, that we have a place in the universe. Whatever we do that is absorbing and soul-nourishing is in *kairos*. Whatever we choose to do from an interior center—from the soul or Self—the greater the likelihood that it will fill us with zest and enthusiasm. Turning toward the soul, we find our internal gyroscope from which we can respond authentically to what is meaningful.

When we realize that we are spiritual beings on a human path, and truly sense that life is a soul journey, it is an internal knowing. It is also a radical shift of perspective from being concerned with what the proverbial neighbors think of us to what really matters to us. Driven by parental expectations, by the need to compensate for low self-esteem, by the internalization of shoulds and oughts, there are high achievers and caretakers who never questioned whether they were doing what they really wanted to be doing with their lives, until a life-threatening illness stopped them in their tracks.

Personal Answers

A life-threatening illness that brings life as usual to a full stop can be soul-serving, if it leads us to develop the inner practice of asking and finding daily answers to these questions:

Are you going to do *something that you want to do,* today? Are you going to spend time doing *something that you love,* today? Are you going to spend time with *someone that you love,* today? Are you going to *follow your instincts,* meandering until you find your spot to be in, today? Are you going to do *work you love,* today? Will there be *beauty in your life,* today? Will you *nourish your soul,* today ? Will *your heart sing,* today?

Recently, I read a short poem by Mary Oliver that provided a picture of how such a day might be. In a few sparse lines, she conveyed spending a day strolling through fields, feeling idle and blessed. She described holding a grasshopper in her hand, and we know she really saw it—as only one who is totally absorbed does. The poem is written as if she were being challenged about how she was spending the day—or is it her life?—so apparently unpurposefully. And yet, it is also clear that she was spending the day being absolutely true to herself, a choice that also honored her understanding of the impermanence of all life. The reader may have begun as a spectator, but the poet cuts through and brings us close to the bone with her last two lines:

> *Tell me, what is it you plan to do*
> *with your one wild and precious life?*[7]

By taking one step at a time, by making one choice at a time, we discover how to know what is authentically true for us. It may begin with how to spend an afternoon and extend to how we want to live and what we want to do with our life, however long or short that might be. Whatever sustains the soul may turn out to sustain and lengthen life as well. By learning how to make choices from within, and acting upon

7. Mary Oliver, "The Summer Day," in *House of Light* (Boston: Beacon Press, 1990), p. 60.

this gnosis of what matters to us, life takes on a sparkle. And if you have a life-threatening illness, and are at a turning point in your life, and if it is to be, health can return as well. These are principles that can be followed, and if they are, I believe that a path will then unfold and lead us home to ourselves, to an inner hearth and a creative fire.

7

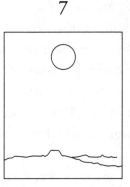

SOMETIMES WE NEED A STORY

Sometimes the difference between life and death begins with a story, especially if the patient has gotten the message that there is no further hope. Expectations are powerful. The words and attitude of others—especially doctors—are potent. They help or hex healing and recovery. When a person is taken into the underworld by a life-threatening illness or a soul-shattering violation, it is an emotional enactment of the myth of the Rape of Persephone. In the beginning, she was gathering flowers in the meadow, and then the earth opened up, and Hades came out of the depths to abduct her.

It was not until Hermes, the messenger god, descended to the underworld and appeared to her, that she realized she would not remain there forever. Hermes, whose Latin name is Mercury, was the god who, with his winged sandals and cap of invisibility, could go between levels and cross boundaries. He was called the guide of souls. When Hermes appeared to Persephone, he brought the message that she could return to the upper world, that recovery was possible.

Hermes is symbolically present in the stories that reach people whose illnesses have taken them into the underworld, to tell them that recovery is possible—especially if they have given up or have been given up by others, and then hear and believe a story that could be about them. Such stories come in many forms. It may be a second opinion sought from another physician; it could be a journal article or information from the Internet, or a story about what someone did to get well, who once was as sick as they are now. These are words that mobilize hope and lead to action; that, in turn, affects the healing response of the body. For words to become a healing story, the message and the messenger must be believed.

I-Thou Physician Bedside Manner

I grew up overhearing my physician mother talking to her patients on the phone. I often heard her ending the conversation with "Don't worry, everything will turn out all right." Whatever a doctor believes and tells a patient is a story that has an effect upon the patient. It has to do with the doctor's "bedside manner," and is part of the art of healing. When physicians with a good bedside manner visit a patient, they don't just review the chart, look at the body part that concerns them, inquire perfunctorily how the patient is doing, and rush out. Even when it is just a matter of minutes, there is an I-Thou quality: the doctor usually looks directly at the patient, and often anchors a comforting or healing message by touch.

This contrasts with the I-It modeling that seems to prevail in medical training settings, where the patient is practically anonymous; rounds are made on "the gallbladder" on the surgical floor or "the M. I." on the cardiac unit. With the proliferation of HMOs, PPOs, and other organizations through which doctors are required to practice assembly-line medicine, matters are worsening for doctors and patients alike. This comes on top of years of advice to practice defensive medicine, which translates into "Don't assure your patient," lest it be considered a verbal contract and grounds for a lawsuit. Instead, increasingly the emphasis is on warning patients of side effects and complications.

When my mother got her medical degree from Columbia University's College of Physicians and Surgeons, sulfa drugs and aspirin were probably the most effective medications that she had to prescribe. She had begun as a G.P., a physician in general practice who delivered babies (later she became a psychiatrist). Bedside manner meant being available, conveying care and concern, and suggesting ways to bring down fevers, and relieve nausea, vomiting, diarrhea, and pain, as well as setting minds at ease with reassurance—while the body usually healed itself. It was second nature for physicians to follow the Hippocratic admonition "Honor the Healing Power of Nature," instead of assuming that they were in charge.

In my psychiatric practice, I know that love for the patient and for the work contributes to my being able to help, something I unexpectedly had confirmed by my "continuous case" in residency. He was a man I saw twice a week for almost two years, and discussed in psychoanalytically oriented supervision once a week. Years later, when I was in private practice, I saw him again, and he said, "You know, what really made a difference was that when you saw me to the door, you smiled at me, no matter what I had said in the session. Your smile told me I was all right." Throughout the session, working as I was with the psychoanalytic model, I maintained neutrality and was, as close as I could be, a blank slate. When the session was over, I was myself as I showed him to the door, and both my optimism and my care for him came through in my smile and voice.

Neutrality can be deadly. When the disease is a metastatic cancer, for example, and the "objective" oncologist tells his or her patient that she is to receive a particular chemotherapy drug with side effects he or she enumerates, which "has a 40 percent chance of being effective," with no discussion or encouragement, the emotional "tilt" is likely more toward hopelessness than hope, on the spectrum of expectations. The patient hears the statistics are not favorable, and surmises: *This isn't likely to help.* The same information presented by an oncologist who has chosen the drug because he or she believes that this particular patient's cancer is likely to be responsive and has positive—or hopeful—expectations, can convey this in his or her words and manner, and this tips the scales toward hopefulness. The patient knows that the doctor cares and has chosen a treatment that he or she believes can help. The statistics are what they are, but the belief becomes: *I can be among those who have a positive response.*

With disease and treatment there is often suffering, discomfort, humiliations, fear, and physical pain. Human beings can endure a lot of suffering for a reason or a cause—for an effort to which they are committed or a story they believe in. It is not suffering in itself that is so hard on the soul; what is deadly is meaningless suffering and feeling powerless to make a difference. Physical and emotional pain are often amplified when such is the case. When suffering is involved, and a course of action might change a critical situation, attitude matters: *If I believe that this might work or that what I am doing matters, I can endure it. If I believe that this will work, it may in fact make it so.*

Recovery Begins with a Positive Emotional Response

What we say and feel as physicians may mean everything to our patients, who often do think the worst about themselves and their condition. Recovery begins with a positive emotional response, a hope or conviction that they can get well that is communicated to the healing system of the body, and the body responds. According to Dr. Candace Pert (who with others published a pivotal paper [1985] in the *Journal of Immunology* called "Neuropeptides and Their Receptors, A Psychosomatic Network"), a psycho-immune-endocrine information network that activates healing is set in motion by the subtle energies of the spirit, and the peptides, which are the information carriers, are released by cells all over the body. In an interview (1995), Dr. Pert elaborated upon this discovery: "Emotions are not in the head. There's a cellular consciousness. There's a wisdom in every cell. Every single cell has receptors on it. The emotional energy comes first, and then peptides are released all over. . . . Consciousness precedes matter. It's not like a peptide creates the feeling. The feeling creates the peptide, on some level."[1]

The Healing Power of a Story

A story has emotional power: it brings meaning, hope, and vision together; it connects body and soul. It can be as simple as a saying or as complex as a biography; it can come from a conversation, a newspaper clipping, a movie, or a myth. A story can bring the power of imagination into a situation. If we identify with the story, it becomes incorporated into us, and every cell and molecule in our body responds. When a person is in a crisis and uncertain, the right words can be life-sustaining. There is an Aha! response when the soul makes a link between *a* story and *my* story, a sense of recognition that something feels intuitively, deeply right; a match between inner inclination and outer configuration. When a patient learns that other patients with this same illness, or the same stage of the illness, recover, it contributes to recovery: if she could or he could do it, *then I can, too!*

When staying alive or recovery depends upon the body's capacity to heal itself, the immune system is involved, and this system is influenced by emotions, images, and thoughts, all of which contribute to a creative imagination that can shape what will actually happen.

The story of "Mr. Wright" and his dissolving tumors is an amazing example of the power of belief and the healing response, in the body of a man with terminal cancer, to that belief. It was reported in the research literature by Dr. Bruno Klopfer[2] and is cited in most contemporary mind-body books.

"Mr. Wright" was the pseudonym for a man suffering from terminal

1. "Candace Pert, Ph.D: Neuropeptides, AIDS, and the Science of Mind-Body Healing," interview by Bonnie Horrigan in *Alternative Therapies in Health and Medicine*, # 1, no. 3 (July 1995), 71–75.
2. Bruno Klopfer, "Psychological Variables in Human Cancer," *Journal of Projective Techniques* 21 (1957): 329–340.

lymphosarcoma. He had "huge tumor masses the size of oranges throughout his body." He had difficulty breathing and required an oxygen mask because his chest was filling with fluid. His cancer had progressed too far for any treatment. Yet, as his physician noted, he clung to the belief that if he were treated with Krebiozen it would cure him. Miraculous cures had been attributed to Krebiozen in the popular press, and he avidly read all he could about this wonder drug.

Coincidentally, Krebiozen was to be tested at the clinic where Mr. Wright was a patient. He did not qualify for the experimental treatment, however: to take part in the trials, a patient had not only to be beyond the reach of standard medical treatment, but to have a life expectancy of at least three months.

Against his better judgment and against the rules of the Krebiozen committee, his physician wrote that Mr. Wright had begged so hard for this "golden opportunity" that he decided that he would have to include him in the trials. The shots were to be given three times a week. The bedridden, gasping Mr. Wright was given his first injection on a Friday. When his doctor returned to the hospital on the following Monday, fully expecting that Mr. Wright might be moribund or dead, he was confronted by a recuperative miracle. Mr. Wright was strolling around the ward, "chatting happily with the nurses and spreading his message of good cheer to any who would listen." Upon examination, the doctor found, in a now-celebrated observation, "The tumor masses had melted like snowballs on a hot stove, and in only these few days, they were half their original size."

Within ten days, Mr. Wright was discharged with nearly all evidence of disease vanished. He was symptom free and even resumed flying his private plane. However, after two months of virtually perfect health. Mr. Wright read that all of the clinics testing Krebiozen were reporting dismal results. He began to lose hope, and relapsed to his former condition.

When he returned to the clinic, his physician made an audacious decision: "Knowing something of my patient's innate optimism by this time, I deliberately took advantage of him. This was for purely scientific reasons, in order to perform the perfect control experiment which could answer all the perplexing questions he had brought up. Furthermore, this scheme could not harm him in any way, I felt sure, and there was nothing I knew anyway that could help him."

Deliberately lying, he told Mr. Wright not to believe what he read in the papers, that the drug was really most promising after all. When the patient logically asked why he had relapsed, he was told that the substance was found to deteriorate on standing, and that a new, super-refined, double-strength product would be arriving the next day. The dissimulations went so far as to delay the fictional shipment's arrival so that his patient's "anticipation of salvation had reached a tremendous pitch."

With much fanfare, and putting on quite an act, the doctor administered an injection consisting of nothing but distilled water. Mr. Wright's second recovery from death was even more dramatic. The masses again melted away, the fluid in the chest vanished, and he became the picture of health until two months later, when the final AMA report came out showing Krebiozen to be worthless. A few days later Mr. Wright came back to the hospital, and within two days of his return was dead.

As I mused about Mr. Wright, I wondered if his cancer could have stayed in remission if he had been told that he had a body with a remarkable ability to heal itself. That it was him, not any magic medicine, that had made the cancer go away, that his story was like Walt Disney's Dumbo and his feather. Dumbo was the little elephant with the enormous ears who couldn't fly until a crow gave him a feather to hold in his trunk and told him it was magic; with it, he could fly. Thinking that the feather made it possible to fly, Dumbo flapped his ears and took off. The feather and a story made it possible for him to do what he had the innate ability to do all along. Knowing that the report on Krebiozen was coming out and that the last injection was water, what if the doctor had told Mr. Wright that, in effect, Dumbo's story was his story?

Krebiozen was tested because claims were made by patients that it had cured them. It was a cancer cure that had been developed by a respected physician whose belief had been substantiated by his results. There were patients to whom he gave Krebiozen, who had had remarkable remissions, and stories about these cancer cures had been reported in newspapers. When clinical trials were done by others, the same substance was injected without the belief of the physician and without the anticipation of a cure by the patient, and was found to be ineffective. The American Medical Association said it was as worthless as distilled water.

That "tumors could dissolve like snowballs on a hot stove" because a man believed he was receiving a miracle drug that could do this is a remarkable story. Not about Krebiozen or about gullibility, but about the remarkable connection between mind and body that is humanly possible, when a patient believes that a miracle cure will cure him, and the healing system of the body does. In his way, "Mr. Wright" had an exceptional talent that went unrecognized.

The reports of other miraculous or spontaneous recoveries substantiate these remarkable healings as within human experience. In 1993, the Institute of Noetics Sciences published *Spontaneous Remission: An Annotated Bibliography,*[3] which was the first survey to report on the phenomenon of remission across the entire spectrum of disease. They documented 430 cases in which the diagnosis was well established and long-term follow-up, where there was little or no allopathic treatment, or where, according to attending physicians, treatment was inadequate—which usually means that medicine had nothing further to offer or would not expect these results from what was done—to account for recovery.

All such cases point to the reality that the body's ability to heal can be mobilized, even after doctors give up. Each case history is a story. Stories that tell us that something is possible *for us* are food for the soul, which in turn influences the mind and body. They also point the way toward what you might do that others have done to enhance your

3. Brenden O'Regan and Caryle Hirshberg, *Spontaneous Remission: An Annotated Bibliography* (Sausalito, Calif.: IONS, 1993).

body's healing response. To do so means exploring possibilities and responding to what makes sense to you and your situation. Belief that you can do something or that something more can be done, when convention says give up and die, changes the course of the journey.

If He Could Do It, Why Can't I?

Elaine Nussbaum was suffering from disseminated uterine sarcoma, a cancer that had spread into her spine and lungs and was not responding to standard medical treatment, when she read an article about a medical doctor, Anthony Sattilaro, who had made a remarkable recovery from metastatic prostate cancer after making major changes in his diet and his philosophy, and something clicked for her.

On April 16, 1980, following eleven months of long and excessive menstrual periods, she'd had a routine dilation and curettage done which had revealed this malignancy. Less than three years later, even after radiation, radical surgery, and aggressive chemotherapy, she had advanced metastatic disease, was confined to a wheelchair, wore a brace, and was in continual pain.

In January 1983 she read about Dr. Sattilaro in a Philadelphia newspaper article that attributed his recovery to macrobiotics. In her book, *Recovery: From Cancer to Health through Macrobiotics,* Elaine Nussbaum recounted her story.

"I thought about macrobiotics, 'It's just food,' I told myself. My knowledge of macrobiotics was very limited, but based on what I already knew, this diet made sense.

"One thought kept recurring. The doctor had been riddled with cancer, and now he was well. 'If he could do it,' I said to myself, 'why can't I?'"[4]

Elaine Nussbaum called the East West Foundation in Brookline, Massachusetts, to get information and begin macrobiotics. With a diet

---

4. Elaine Nussbaum, *Recovery: From Cancer to Health through Macrobiotics* (Tokyo: Japan Publications, 1986; distributed in U.S. by Kodansha International through Harper & Row), p. 130.

prescribed for her condition that was adjusted as she changed, shiatsu massage which was part of the treatment, and a belief that she could get well, Elaine made a decision to stop chemotherapy and follow this alternative treatment exclusively.

She discussed her decision with her oncologist, who agreed to continue to see her regularly. Chemotherapy could be resumed if macrobiotics did not work, but in Elaine's experience to date, chemotherapy had failed to reverse her condition, let alone to stabilize it or to halt the steady progression of the disease. It had made her weak, tired, nauseated, and bald, and reduced her physical mobility and mental clarity. It had caused vomiting, fluid retention, and bone marrow depression, and had depressed her immune system to the point where she had nearly died from a paper cut that became infected.

After two months on the macrobiotic program, instead of getting up to go to the bathroom twelve times a night, she got up only twice. Her stomach was no longer bloated, and she was sleeping better than she had in three years. After three months on macrobiotics, during which she had gradually removed her brace for longer and longer times, she took off the brace for good. She had worn it for eight and a half months. On February 19, 1985, two years after she had begun macrobiotics, Elaine returned to the hospital for a complete set of X-rays of her spine and lungs. There was no cancer in either her lungs or her bones. Three years later, she wrote her book and told her story. At the present time, thirteen years after beginning macrobiotics, she is a macrobiotic counselor herself.

Stories of remarkable recoveries or remissions that are brought about by unconventional means are usually dismissed by conventional medicine as "anecdotal" and ignored. This seems especially so for treatments that support the body's own ability to heal itself, instead of something that is done by a doctor to the body. What medicine also fails to take into account is the complexity and subjectivity of getting sick and getting well, which includes the place that belief itself can play, the need to have reasons to get well, the importance of emotional support, and the power of the doctors' own positive attitude to help the patient (or conversely, for negative expectations to hex the patient).

The psyche is usually left out of the equation, as are any contributions to health that come from non-Western or nonmedical sources—and a remarkable arrogance and ignorance toward such possibilities. Patients increasingly seek alternative therapies and pay out of pocket for them, often while continuing to see their physicians and not telling them. These patients frequently feel forced into making either/or choices without having enough information, and perhaps suspecting, probably accurately, that the alternative therapy they may be rejecting is one that could be of great value.

Soul Companion on a Cancer Journey

In 1991, my friend Patricia had a biopsy done. She had had a mastectomy and chemotherapy for breast cancer with nodal involvement a decade before, and as the years went by, it seemed to be a thing of the past. While we had both been at Cal at the same time years before, our paths hadn't really crossed until we had both been invited to join a women's group. Most of us knew only a few of the others at the beginning, but all of us had in common a spiritual or transpersonal perspective; from there, our friendship had grown. On a pilgrimage in Ireland the year before, Patricia had felt the presence of the goddess in a stone circle meditation that I'd written of in *Crossing to Avalon*. As pilgrims together, I became her soul companion on the journey with cancer that followed.

She had a tumor that I could feel several inches above the reconstructed breast that was the site of the primary cancer. The growth measured about four inches across; it was the size of my palm. It was irregular and firm to the touch and imbedded there. Results of the biopsy brought bad news. It revealed a recurrence of the same cancer, and it was not limited to the tumor. There was no point in excising it, because cancer cells were infiltrating the area. Since it was inoperable or beyond what a surgeon could do, her oncologist recommended Tamoxifen, a chemotherapy drug with an affinity for estrogen-sensitive cancer cells, and a series of radiation treatments. Patricia's diagnosis was not unexpected, and yet it was a total shock, and I saw her alternating between being numb and upset, and thinking matter-of-factly about the reality of the situation and researching both allopathic and alternative treatment choices.

Allopathic medicine uses surgery, chemicals, or radiation to aggressively combat whatever ails the body, while alternative medicine tends to focus on helping the body heal itself, by nutrition, restoring balance, ridding itself of toxins, and engaging the mind and spirit in the process.

Patricia decided that she would take the Tamoxifen and focus on alternatives that strengthen the body's ability to heal itself. She rejected radiation. She looked into the dietary approaches to healing, read widely (including Elaine Nussbaum's book), and made the choice of macrobiotics, which required a major commitment of time, energy, and resources; and she met Nussbaum, who was alive and healthy.

Years before Patricia had this recurrence, I had met O. Carl Simonton, M.D., a radiation oncologist, and been impressed by the effect of his use of visualization on the immune system in the treatment of cancer (I describe this in a later chapter). He maintained that cancer cells—defective, malignant cells—arose routinely in the process of making millions of new cells each day to replace worn-out ones, which our bodies do as a matter of course. However, these bad cells do not normally multiply and develop into cancers, because the body recognizes them as abnormal and rids itself of them. The immune system includes the white cells in the blood and lymph system that come to the body's defense against infections of all kinds as well as cancer. The effect of depression upon the immune system was something I had become familiar with through the University of Rochester's research in psychosomatic medicine, which made a connection between "Giving Up and Given Up" and the development of cancer. The research confirmed that the state of the mind and health of the body are linked—who hasn't been susceptible to "coming down with something" after being physically worn down or depressed?

The macrobiotic course that Patricia had chosen had a philosophical as well as a nutritional basis that focused on enhancing the body's own healing abilities, and I could see and support it as a means of strengthening her immune system. Along with my belief in the connection between mind and matter, and in the possibility of tapping into spiritual sources of healing, I added to her healing process by doing hands-on healing and visualizations with her; she also did visualizations on her own. My prayer group prayed for her, and she was open to what might help her; at the very least, it could not hurt.

Seven months later, most of Patricia's tumor mass had dissolved, and only a hard ridge that felt like thick scar tissue remained. Over the next several months, this too disappeared. When she could detect no signs of the cancer, and she felt healthy and well, Patricia went back to her oncologist for an MRI and a CAT scan, which were normal. There was no evidence of cancer. Maybe this was the result of the macrobiotic diet alone. Maybe it took everything that she did and I did with her, and the Tamoxifen, to bring this about.

Whatever brought about this particular remission began with Patricia's belief that it was possible, which is a soul position. For her, this belief grew out of the stories and experiences of others, and out of her intellectual appreciation of the transpersonal principles and philosophy that underlie macrobiotics. Her mind was solidly behind what she chose to do, and her will kept her on track. From a medical perspective, the remission was remarkable, far beyond what could be expected simply from Tamoxifen.

Stretching Belief to Heal the Body

There were stories I myself drew on that made me able to support Patricia, to believe that what she was doing would work. One was a story that I saw as analogous to what Patricia was doing. I remember when Roger Bannister ran the mile in under four minutes, a feat that was considered physically impossible—faster than humans could run, until he did it. Before Bannister, no one believed it was possible, but once he did it, the belief changed, and from that point on, under four minutes became the norm in world class competition. It seems to me that this same principle applies to healing. Knowing others before you have done it, having the belief that it is possible for you, and doing the equivalent of training, can make it so.

Another story I drew belief from was my own. I'd walked barefoot on a bed of hot coals that had so much heat rising from it I'd had to step back from the edge when I was just watching others do it. Yet when it was my turn, there was no sensation of heat at all as I walked across the same bed of coals. The coals simply sort of crunched under my feet, and I felt as if I were walking on the styrofoam stuff that is used for filler in packing. It was and still is a mystery to me, how this happened. It is in the category of a medical miracle that my skin was unaffected. My mind, however, was unalterably changed. If I could do this, then our bodies are capable of far more than conventional medicine knows.

Case reports of multiple personalities stretched my mind even further about how the body can respond and change. Even though they share the same body, the different personalities can differ physiologically. One can be allergic, while others are not. Eyeglass corrections can differ, as can blood pressure readings and EEGs. When I learned this, it caused me to take a second look at my assumption that we could not own a cat, because cats immediately made my eyes water and itch, and if I didn't leave or take an antihistamine, the reaction would progress until I wheezed and got asthmatic. Medically, I had an inherited predisposition to asthma, hay fever, and atopic dermatitis. But our family dog had died, and now that I had separated from my two children's father, there was no space for a dog. They wanted a cat, and I felt bad that because of my allergy, this was not possible. When I discovered that one multiple personality could be allergic to something that others in the same body were not, then, I reasoned *and believed,* perhaps I could shift out of this allergy.

I was strongly motivated and had decided that after I finished a workshop in southern California near where my mother lives, I would ask her to hypnotize me to get rid of this cat allergy. Meanwhile, I was a houseguest in Malibu, where I had stayed before. Knowing my allergy, my hosts had always made sure that their cat would not come near me. The day I marked as the day I would get rid of this allergy, I awoke to find their cat sitting on my chest facing me. At first I was alarmed and I didn't move, but then I realized that this was *the day,* and here I was sharing breathing space with this cat. I considered this a synchronicity. So we breathed together, face to face, almost touching nose to nose, and I noted that my eyes weren't itchy, that I wasn't wheezing, that something different was happening between me and this cat. After what seemed like quite a long time, the cat moved off me, as if his job were done, and ignored me thereafter, which is how he usually treated strangers. I never did react allergically. I went to my mother's that afternoon, and while I was in a light trance, she suggested I see myself enjoying being nose to nose with the cat again. After that day, it did seem that I was over my cat allergy. The proof of it came when my daughter brought home a cute little kitten who soon became a member of the household.

Bannister's four-minute mile, my experience walking on coals and then overcoming my allergy, these were the stories I told myself. I drew on them to support my own belief that what Patricia was doing for herself, and what I was doing with her, would work. They reminded me of the remarkable effect that mind can have on the body, of what can happen when mind believes and matter conforms to this new belief.

Hermes the Messenger

Information is potent medicine when it is received at the cellular level where soul connects with body. This potent medicine comes in the form of a story that is believed. Metaphorically, these stories are brought by Hermes, the messenger god, who came to tell Persephone that she could return from the underworld, and then brought her back. I feel in my bones that Hermes and neuropeptides are expressions of this communicating link—the messenger—between soul and body. They bring the message that it is possible to heal, or possible to go beyond the conventionally agreed upon physical limits like the four-minute mile, or possible to defy physical laws that bare skin on fiery coals will burn. Just as Hermes brought the message to Persephone and provided the transportation, so it is that when we instinctively believe a healing story, the healing can happen to us.

Whenever there are no definitive cures for a particular illness or stage of it, especially when the disease is AIDS, healing stories may come in the form of experimental allopathic medicine protocols, med-line searches, or alternative approaches. As an example, there is the case of AIDS patient and activist Jeff Getty, who made medical history in December 1995 when he received an infusion of bone marrow cells from a baboon. Jeff finds his healing stories at the cutting edge of medicine.

In an interview in the *San Francisco Chronicle*,[5] Getty was asked what other treatments he had undergone. He responded, "You name it. I have had this disease most of my adult life. I started out really aggressive . . . ," proceeding to name and describe many of the therapies he had undergone. His personal myth prompted him to see himself as "a soldier in the front lines of AIDS, someone willing to die for the cause if necessary, someone willing to take chances." He said, "I was sitting in a foxhole, watching shells landing in my friends' foxholes and watching them die one at a time. I wanted a chance to charge out of my foxhole and fight." Getty could have seen himself as a battlefield on which the war against AIDS was being conducted, but instead he chose an activist role.

Getty and others keep tabs on research and researchers via computer

5. Charles Petit, "A Soldier in the War on AIDS," *San Francisco Chronicle,* January 21, 1996, Sunday Section Interview, pp. 1, 3.

and contacts. When a new possibility arises, they study it thoroughly. During the time of the *San Francisco Chronicle* interview, the transplantation to him of baboon bone marrow tissue had been successfully accomplished, but it was still too early to see the results. He was asked by the reporter, "If this doesn't work, is there anything else you can do besides wait?"

He responded, "I am always on the prowl for something new. One thing I always tell people with HIV is that when you make your plans, always have a backup. So I am looking into the next thing that is out there. For instance, there is something called a thymus transplant, and we are watching that very closely. People with any stage of AIDS, even late-stage AIDS, should remember that as long as you continue to fight and make plans and take actions, you may survive. Some of our friends and I have been, at our lowest points, totally wasted with diseases that we were told would kill us for sure. Well, I am still here."

Getty's "backup" is what I would call another Hermes story— another possibility of healing that he believes might work. To undergo another new treatment and have it fail will not be the end of hope for him, nor will it be meaningless. Staying alive to fight and being part of the AIDS war in and of themselves are sources of meaning for Getty. The treatment efforts he has undergone are not just for himself; they are in service to others because they provide information for the ongoing war. The story he tells himself and believes about what he is doing gives meaning to his struggle. It may very well also prolong his life.

People who involve themselves in their disease and healing have many roles: they are students of the illness and treatments; they are actively involved, not passive patients. They question authority and need physicians who are not threatened by the reality that their patients may have more or newer information than even they do. They are, as many say, enrolled in AIDS University or Cancer U. It is an exacting education, with repeated examinations and constant major tests. And as patients discover—especially if they combine allopathic and alternative treatments, and take the psyche into account—it is a full-time curriculum.

Four years after her second recurrence, some fifteen years after she was first diagnosed with cancer, my friend Patricia's cancer returned for the third time. The choice of what to do *now* again became crucial. Whether it's Jeff or Patricia or you, Hermes is the story that has come for you, the story that tells you that it is possible to return from the underworld into which illness has taken you. These stories have an emotional impact on the soul, and are incorporated and believed at the cellular level. I believe that a person may be drawn to a particular healing story—an allopathic choice, or an alternative choice, or a combination—that may be instinctively right for that person, and not for another. And, as I have seen with my friend, the story—what she needs to do this time—may not be the same story as worked before.

The divine messenger god Hermes could go in either direction; he could go from the upperworld to the underworld, and from the underworld to the upperworld. Mind-to-cell communication must likewise go both ways as well—if a story has an effect on cells, then cells must also influence the instinctive choice of a particular story or choice of treatment, especially if something is nutritionally needed for healing.

In medical school we were told that babies who were weaned and offered a variety of solid foods instinctively chose what their bodies needed. They might eat beets for five days, for example, then switch to something else. However strange their choice of diet, when analyzed nutritionally, the diet made sense. Some of the cravings for particular foods that pregnant women have, and are indulgently mocked for having, also may have to do with nutritional needs or deficiencies, and many of the most effective natural medicines were probably chosen instinctively or, as in the case of an indigenous remedy for an upset stomach, from observing what bears and other animals ate when they were sick.

Humans have animal instincts, *and stories.* Words were carried by Hermes to and from Olympus, the mental realm of the sky and home of divinities, to the underworld where souls dwelled. His words provided guidance to travelers on their journeys. Thus he was the link between realms that represent mind and soul and body. His messenger staff was the caduceus, which has sometimes been confused with the staff of Aesculapius, the symbol of medicine that has one snake. Hermes' staff has two intertwining snakes, an image that reminds me of the double helix strands of DNA that encodes all genetic information at the cellular level.

When stories help to heal us, the stories are archetypal in nature: they are stories that grow out of human experience that have an effect upon us because we share a collective unconscious as described by C. G. Jung. The concept of a human morphic field—the equivalent of the collective unconscious—was put forth by the theoretical biologist Rupert Sheldrake, who maintained that it is our DNA that connects us with what we know in our cells and in the depth of our psyches. Contents of the morphic field or collective unconscious become activated by what we feel and do—by the stories that we believe. There is an allegorical similarity between Hermes and our DNA.

A healing story comes to us like Hermes with his caduceus. The message that recovery is possible, is taken in deeply, heard at the cellular level of our being, and the body responds.

While I was writing this particular chapter, I thought about the ending of my autobiographical book, *Crossing to Avalon: A Woman's Midlife Pilgrimage*. I had used a quote from a children's book called *Crow and Weasel* by Barry Lopez: "If stories come to you, care for them. And learn to give them away where they are needed. Sometimes a person needs a story more than food to stay alive."[6] I meant it figuratively then. Now, I realize that it can be literally true when a person has a life-threatening illness. Sometimes a person really does need a story that provides hope, nourishes the will, or provides meaning, to stay alive.

6. Barry Lopez, *Crow and Weasel* (San Francisco: North Point Press, 1990), p. 48.

8

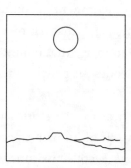

SOUL CONNECTIONS

When the adversity is a life-threatening illness, and the risk is death and/or loss of meaning, an I and Thou relationship to another person is a lifeline and a soul connection. This is especially so when the challenge is to go the distance—to continue on, month after month, with a struggle to get well or to stay alive. In order to keep on keeping on, anyone with an illness that has a long course needs the soul support of others. The daily difficulties and humiliations to do with the wear and tear of physical aches and pains, the mundane and inelegant concern for nutrition and elimination, the fatigue and discouragement that accompanies ill health, the constriction of interests and the limitations that are reminders that you are no longer your old self, take their toll on the spirit.

To keep on keeping on is heroic, and hardly ever acknowledged as such. It is true for the person with the illness and for those who accompany them through the ordeal as well.

When a hard-won period of improvement or remission has raised hopes of recovery, but symptoms return again, it is especially difficult. This happens with any life-threatening condition that took a major toll the first time around. Even when a recurrence or return of symptoms is intellectually expected, people are hardly ever emotionally prepared for it. When there is another serious flare-up of an inflammatory process in an autoimmune disease, or another opportunistic infection with AIDS, or new signs of malignancy, or another heart attack, another stroke, or another almost successful suicide attempt, the recurrence usually ushers in another crisis.

During the initial medical crisis, each experience is new. But subsequent illnesses become increasingly familiar and disheartening. The first time, a patient is like Inanna making a descent through unfamiliar gates, feeling "What is this?" with each new indignity or difficulty. The diagnosis, hospitalization, and treatment are traumatic emotionally, and they are often also physically traumatizing, but all this passes as a necessary part of the process. Once through the ordeal successfully, most painful memories are left behind. But when symptoms return or new signs of disease appear, emotions from the past return as well, sometimes with the impact of a repressed memory. Every cell in the body wants to retract, out of range of a needle or a knife; there is a resistance to going back into a situation that we now know will make us afraid, in pain, nauseated, disoriented, or groggy, not to mention feel little and helpless. It is discouraging to face another round of it, and it takes grit and courage to make the appointments, undergo the tests, and be treated. Who to tell and how they react complicates matters further.

There is also often a sense of shame. Well people may think this bizarre, but almost every chronically sick adult I know who is self-aware knows this to be true. A recurring or a chronic illness is not only difficult to endure physically, but is made doubly difficult psychologically by feelings of being a failure. In our advertising era, when to be beautiful, young, healthy, and affluent is the image against which we are measured, everything and anything that makes us less than that brings shame. People cringe inwardly at the thought of having another bout of illness and at having to put other people through it again. It is this inner reaction, as well as being once more at risk, that is disheartening.

I and Thou Relationships as a Lifeline

In the struggle for health, spirit and soul make a difference. Not to be given up on by others is almost as significant as not giving up on oneself. I-Thou relationships matter, especially when one falters and is caught and kept from plummeting into despair by the heart and hand of another. In this, there are parallels between struggling with a life-threatening illness and a suicidal depression. In a psychiatric practice, the possibility of suicide often arises, and the relationship with the therapist is often the lifeline that keeps patients from killing themselves. When someone is on the cusp between life and death for psychiatric reasons rather than physical ones, the soul issues are clearer, and yet they are the same. Depression and loss of meaning sap body and soul of the will to go on living, when the struggle is so hard.

Early in my office practice, I saw a series of patients who were suicide risks. They were young adults who had been hospitalized at the medical center teaching hospital where I had trained and were considered difficult patients because of their potential to heed self-destructive impulses, their irrational thoughts, and their difficulty forming relationships. They had been discharged on high doses of medication, were often estranged from their families, usually lived in halfway houses, and may have already made suicide attempts. Their lives were difficult and their futures uncertain. All of them were severely self-deprecatory, and if they had auditory hallucinations, the voices were negative and hostile. From time to time, all of them wished that they were dead, and they all had suicidal thoughts. I got emergency phone calls from pay phones on the way to or near the Golden Gate Bridge, as well as many less dramatic yet equally desperate calls. In the midst of an overwhelming wish to die and the possibility of doing something to make it so, the patient would call, reaching out to me to keep from going over the edge. Their relationship with me was their lifeline.

In the beginning years of my private practice, these struggling people were my patients and my teachers. I found myself entering I-Thou two-way conversations with them around issues of living and dying. I abandoned the psychiatric stance of neutrality, of being a blank screen, or reflecting back what the patient was saying. It was in these conversations that I intuitively felt that at the soul level—beyond what the ego knows or can define—they recognized the truth was being spoken; when another person's life is on the line, only honesty and honest hope will do.

If one person is a lifeline for another during a crisis, it is because love and respect exist for the person and for the struggle. At a time when the light in the other is faltering, the message that "You matter" and "This struggle has meaning," encoded in a soul-to-soul connection—with or without being explicitly said—is the lifeline. When the threat to life is suicide, and the suffering is psychological, the effort to keep on keeping on, is different, and yet in some existential way it is similar to the toll on the spirit that comes from a recurrent or chronic physical illness. The soul-to-soul connection with another, an I-Thou friend, therapist, or partner, can make the difference between giving up and going on.

What We Know in Our Bones

What we believe or feel in our bones are matters to do with soul. We can voice such beliefs, and when we do, there is a possibility we will be heard and responded to, because this level of belief is archetypal. For example, I cannot persuade you with logic that we are spiritual beings on a human path, but just saying this may articulate what you know in your bones is so. Words that bring us close to the bone may be philosophical restatements of perennial wisdom or they may be homespun sayings that strike a deep note, and become words to live by from childhood onward.

Words that I heard when I was growing up that stuck with me and provided a perspective for the unfairness and suffering I encountered were "Everyone has a cross to bear," and "We are not given more to carry than we can bear." Even without much life experience, I felt there was truth in these sayings. At the same time, my mind wondered if they were true, and I began to check them out. In high school and college, I had only to know someone well, to see behind the carefree or privileged facade that they otherwise presented to the world. Often, even decades before the concept of dysfunctional family, to know someone well was to know about the pain they had in their family. Everyone I knew well seemed to have "a cross to bear." To believe that we are not given more to carry than we can bear takes more faith—or an awareness that this is so for individual souls, who accept the trials of life as theirs to live well.

I was reminded of this when I heard about the life and death of a woman who had died at thirty of cystic fibrosis. Her friend Martha, who told me her story, described her as an ebullient soul, someone "who did not let the dark cloud over her life dim her bright spirit." She had refused a lung transplant, saying she wanted to keep the organs she was born with. She accepted her lungs as they were, as she had accepted her life with cystic fibrosis as her fate; but acceptance was not resignation. She was an example to her friend, of someone "who truly lived her karma," which is another way of seeing life from a spiritual perspective. She continually had pushed the envelope, not only exceeding her life expectancy but doing things that were extraordinary for someone with this disease. She had accepted the challenge to live her predictably foreshortened life fully, and she had lived it well.

When I heard about her, words from T. S. Eliot's *Four Quartets* came to my mind. I have toted copies of the *Four Quartets* around with me for decades, and consider it a theology of the Self, whose enigmatic words make sense; when they do, it is said perfectly, which is to say that the words are distillates of wisdom and image that come together when understood, mind and soul. In this case, the words echoed the reality of a shortened life lived fully and beautifully against a backdrop of the eternal: "The moment of the rose and the moment of the yew-tree / Are of equal duration."[1]

1. Eliot, "Little Gidding," *Four Quartets*, lines 232–233.

*

Martin Buber, the philosopher-theologian, coined "I-Thou" as an expression of a quality of relationship, an intimacy on a soul level, that immediately is grasped by anyone who has had such a relationship— with another person, or mystically with a divine presence. From the psychological perspective of C. G. Jung, an I-Thou relationship is one in which the Self is constellated or felt: We have a subjective perception that this experience has meaning; we tap into a spiritual source or wellspring. I-Thou is about love and intimacy and trust between two souls, or a soul and divinity.

Life-Threatening Illness as a Spiritual Journey

From the standpoint of the soul, a life-threatening illness is a spiritual journey—an adventure or an ordeal or an initiation—that is undertaken by the patient and can be shared by others. The possibility of losing a sense of meaning as well as losing life are risks for the patient and her companions; the possibility of finding one's soul and living or dying within an I-Thou relationship is the opportunity for both. For anyone else in the emotional vicinity of another's life-threatening illness, there are choices of how to respond that may have spiritual consequences for that person. When there is a delicate balance between living and dying at this point in the patient's life, an I-Thou companion may make the difference between survival and death.

A life-threatening illness that happens to someone close to us, takes us into the underworld as a companion on the journey, and inasmuch as it will take us into our own depths of feeling and meaning, there are consequences for us as well.

An illness that happens to someone close to us can bring us close to the bone, to the essence of who we are and what we are here for at a soul level. It is not just the patient but others who are tested by illness. When the life that is threatened or the body that is failing is not ours, it still affects us deeply; it can become a soul experience for us. If we are spiritual beings on a human path, and we encounter a life-threatening illness on that path, the same questions arise for patient and potential companion: in this life and in this situation, what did we come to do? what did we come to learn?

When anyone is in big trouble or a personal disaster strikes, everyone else in the emotional vicinity is affected and has a reaction to the news. It is a moment of truth, a telling moment, that says volumes. There are conscious decisions or automatic responses, to move toward or move away from that person. It may be news of a life-threatening illness, but it could as well be about any major trouble that happens to people: a mental illness, a rape or assault, a suicide attempt, financial or legal trouble, loss of a relationship through death or divorce, anything really difficult that is part of life that we don't want to happen to us. When I learn that someone in my emotional vicinity is having a hard time, is sick, may be dying, or is dying, will my friend, spouse, relative have to face this alone? Or will someone be there—*really be there?* Will it—can it—be me?

Moments of Truth

The diagnosis of a life-threatening illness is a moment of truth for the well ones. Regardless of the degree of commitment before the diagnosis, after the diagnosis, what it means to be committed *now,* will present itself *over and over.* Viktor Frankl's lesson to us—that regardless of circumstance, we have a choice of how we will respond—has enormous applications for the person who accompanies another on this part of the journey, *or* moves away from her or him. Emotional distancing is a common reaction, and actual abandonment also happens.

Fear of loss and fear of abandonment are what keep us from being fully ourselves with others. What happens in us then, when we know someone who matters to us may die or is dying? Or when an illness has progressed to where we know someone we love *is* leaving us. Do we draw back? Or do we draw near? Do we enter a deeper relationship at an I-Thou level, or do we leave them emotionally or physically before they leave us?

As spiritual beings on a human path, relationships present us with the greatest opportunity to grow and learn, and the greatest potential to be psychologically wounded and then to act defensively or in retaliation, hurting others and damaging ourselves at a soul level. It matters how we respond. We cannot treat another person shabbily without that shabbiness sticking to us; we cannot respond generously without our hearts expanding and nourishing the soul.

It is a risk to be authentic and shed persona, armor, defenses; and it is a loss if we do not take the risk, for then there is no possibility of intimacy. If we live behind gates emotionally, thinking that this will keep us safe, the only certainty is that our decision will keep us isolated, in a box of our own making. Especially when an illness if life-threatening, and we have the opportunity either to have a meaningful exchange or a meaningless one, will we seize the moment or let it pass, even if this may be the last chance we have for an I-Thou connection with this particular person? In relationships, there is risk in venturing out beyond the gates, and risk in remaining guarded; saying something or saying nothing may be equally crucial to them and to us.

When we want to say something that is on our heart about ourselves or about the other person, to that significant person, the words are just behind our lips: will we open our mouth and let them out, or will we swallow the words and wait for another time? How prickly is the other person? How sensitive or defensive are we? How safe is it? Will this make matters better or worse? Will we be understood or judged? Will there be tears or anger? What has our experience been in the past? Can we be vulnerable with no guarantees?

No wonder people have been compared to porcupines, who need to get close to each other for warmth, but never too close.

These are the questions that are always present in relationships. But when we also have to take a serious illness into account, we become aware of something that actually is *always* so: The present moment may be a now-or-never moment.

Relationships Enter a Crucible

When a life-threatening illness intrudes on ordinary life, the usual relationship patterns also shift. Significant relationships enter a crucible, where they are heated and stressed; cracks appear when bonds are flawed and break, then people distance themselves emotionally or leave. Or the opposite occurs: bonds of love become stronger, more flexible, and more beautiful, as if shaped and burnished by difficult events that reveal more and more soul.

It is in the eyes and hearts of others that we see our own reflections. When appearance matters and status matters and has mattered to others around us, beginning with our parents, it's difficult to know whether we intrinsically matter to anyone. When our health goes, we neither look good nor perform well. Then what? This is when the alchemy of relationships takes people into the crucible. Will the sick person withdraw into herself or himself, and not allow anyone to come close? Will the healthy person leave, emotionally or physically?

When physical attractiveness or having a position of power and prestige were essentials in forming the relationship in the first place, a serious illness tests the relationship even more. Beauty, vitality, and youthfulness require good health, as does staying on top in a competitive field. When it's no longer possible to be or do what made us attractive initially, will the relationship die before the patient does? Will the illness be the means for both individuals to discover a depth of soul and love that they did not know was possible? Illnesses that take away physical attractiveness also strip away emotional defenses such as the illusion of being in control, of invulnerability, or of eternal youth for both the patient and partner. The onset of such an illness presents a challenge for the individual and for the couple: A time to grow up and grow deeper presents itself.

In Tony Kushner's Pulitzer Prize–winning play, *Angels in America,* there are several powerful scenes that focus on the relationship between the healthy partner (Louis Ironson) and his lover (Prior Walter), who has AIDS. Before Louis leaves Prior, he tells a nurse about the Bayeux Tapestry, which leads him to fantasize about the difference between La Reine Mathilde, who embroidered the tapestry, and his own reaction to Prior's illness:

> Mathilde stitched while William the Conqueror was off to war. She was capable of . . . more than loyalty. Devotion.
>
> She waited for him, she stitched for years. And if he had come back broken and defeated from war, she would have loved him even more. And if he had returned mutilated, ugly, full of infection and horror, she would still have loved him; fed by pity, by a sharing of pain, she would love him even more, and even more, and she would never, never have prayed to God, please let him die if he can't return to me whole and healthy and able to live a normal life. . . . If he had died, she would have buried her heart with him.
>
> So what the fuck is the matter with me?[2]

"Louis" exists as a disloyal voice in spouses and lovers of patients with any life-threatening, debilitating, or chronic illness. "Louis" is afraid and untested; his partner's illness calls on him to face his fears and his shadow, to be and do more than he knows how. "Louis" runs instead of staying, which is what happens when the Louis part of a person prevails.

"Louis" idealizes "Mathilde," and doesn't know that becoming "Mathilde" doesn't happen overnight or easily, but is a result of responding to each new situation with an action or an attitude, through which one grows by being a soul companion to an ill or dying person. What "Louis" also doesn't know is that love transforms the person into someone who continues to be able to love, after the loss; the heart—or capacity to love—is not buried with the death of the loved one.

When sacrifices are willingly made, they are made from the heart—

2. Tony Kushner, *Angels in America*, part 1: *Millennium Approaches*, act 2, scene 3 (New York: Theater Communications Group, 1992, 1993), pp. 51–52.

not from fear or obligation. It is a choice that is rewarded with soul growth, a sense of inner strength, and a firsthand knowledge of love. It may look like codependency or martyrdom or victimhood to someone else, who doesn't know better, but it isn't that when a choice to love and be there has been made. When love and loyalty are the reasons for remaining devoted to someone who is ill, and the response to whatever happens is to do whatever is called for, the journey may turn out to be a spiritual path, with unexpectedly rich soul moments.

I have known this to happen in men whose partners had AIDS or whose wives had cancer, who opened their hearts and were devoted in ways that I previously only knew to be women's experiences. Gay men, especially, have made a quantum soul leap in the AIDS epidemic. Relationship is a spiritual practice under these circumstances, and daily, repetitious, and mundane tasks are the daily devotions through which a lover, spouse, or friend expresses unconditional love. There is happiness when for a time, all is well, or better than it was. Great tenderness unlike anything known before wells up in unexpected moments; looking at a sleeping face warms the heart. And there is gratitude.

Mutuality Even When One Is Ill and the Other Is Well

When two individuals are present for each other in heart, mind, and soul while one is going through the travails of a possibly fatal illness, it is an I-Thou relationship, and an opportunity for emotional and spiritual intimacy of the highest order. For this, both need to be committed to each other and to believe that the passage is a significant one for both. While it may seem that it is the healthy partner who must make the choice to go deeper, to have the other matter more, it is as difficult a challenge for the person with the life-threatening illness.

An I-Thou relationship calls upon *both* to love more, now. It calls upon the person with the illness to be concerned for the other, and not focus entirely on herself or himself, at a time when fear and pain make self-absorption easy. To truly share the journey requires being present, being real, and being vulnerable together through this scary passage. The interior struggle between love and fear is accentuated by having a life-threatening illness or by loving someone who has one. For the ill person to express words of love and want assurances of love in return, especially while feeling increasingly less attractive, is a risk. Or the risk may be in wanting to be touched but not wanting to be sexual, and voicing it. Or there may be a need for solitude, and fear of being rejecting to speak of it. Or questions that lie on the heart; will they be asked and answered?

Anger, resentment toward the other, and fear about the other arise in both people, when one of them has a life-threatening illness and the other is healthy. Of course this is so, for both are vulnerable, often short of sleep, and often worried about the other people and matters affected by this crisis, as well as by the illness itself. It is a scary but precious time, through which I-Thou relationships can form or grow.

Soul Connections

When the possibility of death arises, relationships with people and with God become more intense. Priorities shift, facades drop away, and the need for meaning and soul connections becomes acute, all of which affect relationships. A soul encounter or soul moment on a particularly significant part of a path can make the difference between going on or giving up. In the Himalayas, as travelers pass each other on the mountain, they bow or nod to each other and say, *"Namaste,"* which translates into "The divinity in me beholds the divinity in thee." Whenever two individuals meet on the path that is the metaphor for life, and there is a soul-to-soul moment, this is the underlying and unsaid greeting. *"Namaste"* acknowledges the I-Thou.

There are I-Thou moments and I-Thou companions. I-Thou companions are at times side by side as well as face to face; they also can be back to back, so to speak, when guarding the back of the other. For two people to be soul companions, the relationship has to be a *temenos* or sanctuary, where it is safe to be oneself, to be unguarded, to trust that *this vessel can hold the contents.* The vessel is more than the love between the two people, though love between the two is an essential ingredient.

For a relationship to be a sanctuary, in principle it must be safe to tell the truth of what you feel, think, and perceive; in practice this is an ongoing process that requires risk and trust and time, because we all enter relationships with secrets and vulnerabilities. The possibility of disillusionment for either when you take a risk, the wish for closeness and fear of engulfment which both may have in different proportions, the various defenses and denials that operate unconsciously, and the hurt that results when there is an inevitable discrepancy between our expectations of each other and reality makes an I-Thou union a major undertaking. In that such relationships call upon our capacity to love, to forgive, to speak the truth, and to act upon the truth as we perceive it, and keep faith makes a relationship a spiritual path in itself.

A soul connection may be the key to a remarkable recovery, which defies conventional medical expectations. In their study of people who made remarkable recoveries, Caryle Hirshberg and Marc Ian Barasch described their findings under "social connections," while I think of such relationships as "soul connections" in which both the patient and the significant other person or inner figure is in an I-Thou relationship. Hirshberg and Barasch wrote: "People in their lives often 'came through' in the moment of crisis—or else new friends and allies surfaced to support them on their journey. Even those who attributed their recoveries to powerful inward experiences seemed to feel a deep personal connection with the imagined figures or spiritual presence they encountered."[3]

Hirshberg and Barasch noted, "Time after time, we saw the power of enduring marriages, devoted friendships, selfless acts, and indestructible love. One well-chosen utterance, one strongly conveyed belief, one palpable gesture from a friend or loved one often provided the hand that pulled someone from the abyss."

3. All references to Hirshberg and Barasch are taken from Caryle Hirshberg and Marc Ian Barasch, *Remarkable Recovery* (New York: Riverhead Books, 1995).

The significant relationship that made a difference might not have even been in the patient's life before the diagnosis: "Patients often forged unusually strong relationships with a doctor, a therapist, a friend, or a support group. Over and over, we were struck by 'the power of one'—how just one person's encouragement in the struggle against the most horrendous odds formed the pivot of healing, and how one remarkable recovery often rippled outward to inspire others—and sometimes, to affect society at large."

Circles of Support

I-Thou relationships also occur within a circle of people who create a *temenos* where it is safe to speak about what really matters, and all are committed to listen with compassion. Such a circle is a healing environment that not only supports the emotional well-being of its members but, especially when it is a cancer support group, extends life as well.

This was first reported as an unexpected research finding by David Spiegel, M.D., a professor of psychiatry at Stanford University, who had begun a study in the mid-1970s involving eighty-six women with metastatic breast cancer. He wanted to see "if a psychosocial intervention would help women with breast cancer cope more effectively with the particular types of fear and isolation that they frequently came to experience."[4] To study this, women with similar characteristics and diseases, all of whom were receiving standard medical treatment, were randomly selected to be in a support group, or not. As a standard against which change could be measured, those who were not in a support group would be compared with those who were; they formed the control group. The women in the support group came to care very deeply for one another. Besides sharing what they were going through and talking about death and dying, radiation and chemotherapy, pain and disabilities, they supported each other in realigning priorities and social

4. David Spiegel, "A Psychosocial Intervention and Survival Time of Patients with Metastatic Breast Cancer," *Advances: The Journal of Mind-Body Health,* vol. 7, no. 3 (Summer 1991), p. 12.

networks, in communicating with doctors, in sharing information and experiences about alternative treatments. These women were encouraged to develop a life project, to accomplish something important to them in the time they had left. There was also a monthly meeting with family members, and training in self-hypnosis for pain management.

Spiegel and his associates measured mood disturbances and pain experiences, and established that women in support groups did significantly better than those in the control groups. They published their results and forgot about the study for a few years. Then, provoked by claims about the power of the mind to cure cancer, which he thought to be foolish, Spiegel returned to his original study assuming that he would be able to show that being in a support group had had no effect on the progression of the disease. What he found astonished him: the women in support groups had survived twice as long as those who were in the control group. At the ten-year point in 1989, they had lived an average of 36.6 months, while the participants in the control group, who had received standard medical treatment alone, survived an average of 18.9 months. Furthermore, three women who had been in support groups were still alive.

From my experience in women's circles, I know that when trust is established, circles become a growth medium. Women have a powerful effect on each other in safe groups, seeing themselves reflected back by the responses of others. They have a remarkable capacity to exhibit strength one moment and vulnerability the next. In a circle, each woman is a unique person; she is herself and yet she is also an aspect of every other woman in the circle. We express emotions, cheer each other on, hug one another, laugh and cry together. We celebrate occasions, rituals that honor the small and large passages, the personal accomplishments, and events that we have learned matter. What happens to one reverberates greatly in the psyches of the others.

In support groups, there is a sharing of specific information when it might be helpful, names of people, articles, tapes, books, helpful hints, even recipes. I assume that women being women, Spiegel's groups were similar to those I am familiar with. In a cancer support group, they would share what they were doing and learning about their cancers.

People who have come through surgery, radiation, chemotherapy, transplants, hormones, dialysis—the varied sometimes effective and often painful or difficult tools of modern medicine—have made it through extraordinarily challenging personal ordeals. That there is an analogy between this and mountain climbing helped inspire the expedition comprised of survivors of breast cancer, to make the 23,000-foot climb of Mt. Aconcagua, the highest peak in South America. This expedition had as its motto: "No one ever said the fight to end breast cancer would be a walk in the park." To make such climbs, individuals are roped together. If one should slip, the others can break the fall. The rope is a lifeline when this happens, and success depends upon team effort. Where one person climbing alone might fall to her death or one woman struggling alone with breast cancer might give up, the bond or lifeline to others makes survival possible. Such is the importance of I-Thou connections in support groups.

People with AIDS and those close to them have similar feelings of sharing a struggle, though the commonest metaphor is one of living in the midst of a plague while others go on with life as usual, unaware of the struggles all around them.

The combination of intention, will, time, and commitment creates the space or the vessel—for grace to enter, for love to be present, or for one soul to touch another, even if it is in the context of a research project. I-Thou moments bridge our separateness and heal the loneliness brought on by separation and isolation from each other and from divinity. These moments heal the soul and in turn have an effect on the body. Quality of life is enhanced, and life itself is extended.

Soul Links

I and Thou moments can also occur in silence. I think of a woman who described sitting at the bedside of her father, who had Alzheimer's disease. She had only known him previously as an emotionally distant, physically abusive, angry man whom she had either feared or hated, and now felt obligated to visit. But at some point, the fear left over from her childhood dissipated, and she felt an upwelling of compassion for him. She reached out and placed her hand lovingly over his and sat in silence with him, feeling peace pass between them. Even though his mind was gone—maybe even because it was gone—the essence of him was still there, and she felt a soul link. Thereafter, she visited regularly and would sit in a meditative silence with him, feeling each time that they were meeting at a soul level. For the remainder of his life, she visited regularly and continued to feel this bond. I didn't doubt her perception that she now had a relationship with her father, a beautiful one. And I also agreed with her speculation that his mind and character armor had to go for this to have happened. Her experience led me to suggest this possibility to others, that rather than give up when a parent or partner was not herself or himself anymore, it still might be possible to be with the essence of the person, to meet on a soul level.

Inanna and Persephone: Myths of Recovery

When a person has been abducted into the underworld of physical or mental illness, and there is even a remote possibility of returning to the land of the living, a bond with another person who has not given up on her or him may make all the difference. As in mythology, without Ninshubur, Inanna's loyal friend, Inanna could never have returned to the upperworld.

Without Demeter, Persephone would have remained in the underworld, but Demeter did not give up. First she searched for nine days and nine nights and couldn't find Persephone anywhere. Then she learned that Persephone had been abducted by Hades with Zeus's permission, and was told she might as well adjust to this; what had happened was beyond her power to prevent and apparently beyond her power to change. However, as the myth tells us, Demeter refused to accept the loss as final. While Persephone remained in the underworld, her mother suffered. She was initially frantic and was unable to eat, sleep, bathe, or care for her appearance. Demeter was angry about what had happened, and then tried to sublimate her loss by taking care of another woman's child. When this didn't work, she withdrew into her temple, depressed, and as a result, nothing on earth grew.

When Demeter was told about Persephone's abduction, it was like being given a diagnosis and a prognosis, with the assumption that she would, of course, accept them. Her daughter was in the realm of death and would not return. Likewise, Ninshubur had been told by the first two gods she'd appealed to on Inanna's behalf, "Give up, no one returns from the underworld."

But because neither gave up, we have myths of return that parallel recoveries from illness, especially those recoveries that depend upon a soul connection. In these stories, a person returns from the underworld of illness because another does not give up. At a soul level, I believe that subtle lines of connection—of love—can provide sustenance for the spirit to stay in the body. People survive when medical authority has no expectations of survival, simply because they do not let go of life; they may barely hang on, as one might to a ledge, with their fingertips, but they hang on rather than leave the other behind. Recovery becomes possible because someone who loves you refuses to give up, or perhaps it is someone in you who refuses to give up.

Demeter and Persephone can personify a parent (especially a mother) and a sick or dying child. They can represent the connection between two adults, when one is well and the other is at risk of dying. For the person who is "Demeter" not to give up may make the difference between life and death. "Persephone" is in the underworld, and the possibility of dying is real, but Demeter's refusal to abandon Persephone to her fate makes recovery possible.

Demeter and Persephone can also represent two aspects of the person who is sick and in the midst of a life-threatening illness. When anyone is really sick and the body is wasted, Persephone, as the symbol of health and vitality, is gone. Recovery depends upon her return. Not to give up on yourself is to feel and look like grieving Demeter, but like Demeter, not to give up in spite of what you have been told is to identify with the myth and believe, without knowing how, that health will return.

Soul connections are life sustaining when there is a danger from succumbing to a descent. Being held in the consciousness of another person matters. Being prayed for does. One devoted person waiting for another to emerge from anesthesia or from a coma can be why someone with a tenuous connection to life does return.

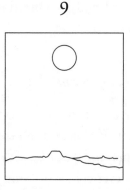

9

SUMMONING ANGELS: PRAYER

W hen we pray for someone, an angel goes to sit on his shoulder." Pat Hopkins, who coauthored *The Feminine Face of God,* came up with this image in a discussion on prayer, and it has stayed with me as an apt description—not only of what I hope happens when I pray, but as a metaphor for the summoning and sending of invisible support.

When we are most vulnerable or desperate for ourselves or for others, we pray. When we, or someone we love, have a life-threatening illness, we pray. When our survival or the survival of someone we love depends upon surgery or other drastic measures, we pray. When we or someone we love is beyond cure, still we pray. In prayer we reveal our fears and hopes and need for help, we focus on what really matters to us, we pray about matters that we have otherwise kept to ourselves. Praying can heal our isolation, strengthen our ability to keep on keeping on, and nourish our spirit. When we pray, we tap into a divine mystery and source, call upon a relationship with something greater than ourselves. We seek and find a connection between ego and Self, between ourselves and God.

Angels and Prayer

Prayer is a way of holding others in my consciousness in a positive way, in a way that worry cannot. When a fear for someone crosses my mind, my response is a one-line prayer: "Please be with him," or "Keep her safe," or "Comfort them," whatever comes to mind. I don't want to add my own fear and worry to the dark cloud of fear the person I'm afraid for no doubt already feels or generate fear for someone who is unaware of danger. Better to send angels to spread their protective wings around them.

When I pray for myself or for others, I notice that it centers me, that there is a quieting of the noise that my mind makes, that I am absorbed in the present moment. I often have a sensation—a slight ache or pressure—in the center of my chest when I pray, in an area that would be covered by my hand, if I placed the heel of my hand upon my sternum and between my breasts. Sometimes when I pray, I put my hand there. It's as if there is a physical correlation to opening my heart as a receptive and perceptive organ of consciousness, when I pray and quiet comes.

Maybe this is what letting an angel in or out feels like, or breathing an angel into the heart feels like. Maybe an angel is a quantum of serenity that enters and fills us when we pray. Or goes to surround those we pray for. Maybe an angel's protective wings are energy fields, a sanctuary in the midst of fearful situations. Maybe when angels watch over us, healing is facilitated. Maybe we are the angels and healing energies are extensions of the love that we send when we pray or touch with the intention of comforting or healing.

Healing Effect of Prayer

While we have only our subjective feelings to support the practice of prayer as having an effect, the belief that we are doing something for people with life-threatening illnesses when we pray is supported by research. Larry Dossey, M.D., assembled the scientific evidence of the healing power of prayer in his book *Healing Words: The Power of Prayer and the Practice of Medicine.* The research done at San Francisco General Hospital by cardiologist Richard Byrd was especially noteworthy.

Over a ten-month period, a computer assigned 393 coronary care unit patients to either a group that was prayed for by home prayer groups (192 patients) or to a group that was not prayed for (201 patients). They were randomly selected to be in each group in this double-blind experiment. None of the patients, nurses, or doctors knew which group any of the patients were in. Byrd recruited various religious groups to pray for the patients in the prayed-for group, who were given the first names of the patients and a brief description of their conditions and diagnoses. Each person prayed for many different patients, and each patient in the experiment had between five and seven people praying for him or her.

The results were impressive: The prayed-for patients were five times less likely to require antibiotics (three versus sixteen patients); they were three times less likely to develop pulmonary edema (six versus eighteen); none of them required an artificial airway and a mechanical ventilator (zero versus twelve), and though this is not statistically significant, fewer patients who were in the prayed-for group died.[1]

In my mind, there are people with life-threatening illnesses whose life-or-death fate seems to teeter precariously. With them, one thing may tip the scales. The illness may have begun with an infection; a chemical shift or a cellular change; repressed anger, hopeless despair; a depletion of physical, psychological and spiritual resources; environmental toxins; a genetic susceptibility; or a combination that added up

1. Larry Dossey, *Healing Words: The Power of Prayer and the Practice of Medicine* (San Francisco: HarperSan Francisco, 1993), pp. 179–81. Original study by Randolph C. Byrd, "Positive Therapeutic Effects of Intercessory Prayer in a Coronary Care Unit Population," *Southern Medical Journal* 81:7 (July 1988): 826–29.

to disease. My own intuitive speculation is that there are not only crucial moments but months, or even years, during which the outcome of
most diseases can be reversed. Besides standard medical treatment, it
cannot hurt to pray for healing, since there are no adverse side effects.
I think that a prayer can sometimes be like a feather on a delicate scale
that tilts the process in the direction of health, especially if a loss of
spirit is contributing to the illness.

When we pray for ourselves or someone else, we may in effect be
sending an angel to help—as we are asking or inviting an interaction
between the invisible world and the physical one. Since humans cannot
really know what God is or know what an angel is, even after a lifetime
of worship or a life predicated on the existence of God, what we are
effecting when we pray is in the realm of faith and speculation. However, as Dossey's book notes, the effects of prayer can be substantiated
by research. Whether we affect the mind of God by prayer, or shift an
archetype, or activate a morphic field, there *is* something we effect
when we pray.

"Dear God / Goddess / Spirit / Powers greater than my small self"

As real and as personal as prayer is to me, I have had the irreverent
thought of beginning with "To whom it may concern." The words and
form that humankind has used to address prayers to divinity change
from culture to culture and over time. Prayers have been directed—and
still are—to gods and goddesses, animal and spirit powers, saints or
ancestors, as well as to the monotheistic male God of Judeo-Christian
tradition. Regardless of who or what is addressed, a belief in the existence of divinity to whom we are related is innately human.

In our bones, we have a sense of the sacred, of a relationship to a
power greater than ourselves that is archetypal and prehistorical. What
does it matter, really, how we pray? I am reminded of a man who told
me how he'd gotten over a major problem for him, of "who" to address
his prayers to, when he hit bottom as an alcoholic. He was an agnostic
with an intellectual awareness of the many gods worshipped by humans

over the millennia and the many atrocities done in the name of divinity. In his bottomed-out state, his crisis was life threatening, and he knew that his only hope was to call upon a higher power, yet he blocked when it came to how to address his prayers. The solution that finally worked for him was to address them to every divinity he thought of by name, and to call upon dead spiritual teachers or holy people as well.

People ordinarily think that prayer is through words, with silent prayers ones that are not said out loud. But this is a limiting description of prayer. Men and women with religious vocations, especially those in contemplative orders, shift into a prayerful state of being. There are many ways of praying, and many postures that can accompany prayer. When divinity is defined and experienced as God above, physical posture while praying reflects this, as well as words. Yet even this is not always obvious. To prostrate oneself before God, which is to lie on one's face with arms outstretched in humility, looks very much like the position taken by a woman who lies upon the earth, as Alice Walker does, to be comforted and strengthened by contact with the earth itself, by Mother Earth, goddess.

Prayer Expressed Through the Body

Dance and song in many cultures is prayer. A decade ago, I first appreciated how this could be so when I watched my friend Arisika Razak, a dancer and a black midwife, perform. It was the first time that I had seen dance that was both sensual and sacred. I was witnessing prayer expressed through the body, dance as ritual, choreographed movement that was as archetypal as giving birth. When she danced, it was a body prayer in which Arisika was Woman and Priestess, and an expression of the Goddess.

As I described in *Crossing to Avalon,* I have gradually come to know that divinity is both transcendent—as God—and embodied—as Goddess—and that it is through women that the energy of the goddess most naturally flows. The first I-Thou moment that everyone comes into the world ready to receive is through touch, not words. A woman who gazes with love and wonder at her infant in her arms is, at that moment, an embodiment of the madonna and child. Women often experience these moments as sacred, as times in which both were surrounded by peace, by an aura which medieval artists captured as a golden halo.

Healing Touch

At the end of life as at its beginning, a woman may act as midwife, only this time as midwife to the soul as it crosses the threshold. Held in the arms of a woman, or more rarely by a man whose interior feminine allows him access to the mother archetype, a dying person may feel himself or herself held by the Mother, embraced by an energy that surrounds both, participating in a prayer without words, receiving unconditional love through the body of the woman as the conduit.

Prayers are healing words. Healing touch is also prayer. Years ago, when my children were little, and either of them were "coming down with something," I would sit on the edge of their beds, and put the palm of my hand or both hands over what was not well, and be with them. I prayed that love would flow through me, through my arms to my hands and into them, and that they would get well. It was hardly a controlled experiment, but it did seem that beginning sore throats and beginning chest colds did get better, and they were rarely sick in childhood. It felt good because I was doing something that might help. To share this kind of prayerful moment is to be in a meditative field together, linked by physical as well as spiritual contact.

I think that anyone who does hands-on healing begins with an awareness of being filled with compassion for the sick person: this fullness of love, like priming a pump, allows us to draw from a deeper, transpersonal, upwelling source. Healing then flows through our heart and hands to the other person, as a subtle and powerful energy.

I tell other people what I do so they might try it. I believe that all of us have innate healing abilities, that love is the energy that heals, and that this conduit requires only that we open a channel to it, and direct it by our focus. This is the same principle as prayer for others, or for ourselves, to open the heart, and let it fill with love and peace, and then direct it—this time through our hands to a person who needs healing.

Therapeutic Touch

What I did with my children was a "homey" version of laying on of hands. Therapeutic Touch, introduced into nursing by Dolores Krieger, professor of nursing at New York University, and now used by nurses in hospitals, hospices, and in home care, is a contemporary method of laying on of hands with a theoretical basis in physics and in Eastern concepts of *prana* or *qi* energies. A nurse practitioner begins by centering herself, quieting her mind, and becoming meditative and receptive. Then, she uses her hands to scan the body of her patient, a few inches above the skin, assessing or sensing disturbances in the energy field. Then, with her hands still above the skin, she works at rebalancing the energy field around the patient, smoothing out knots of tension, directing healing energy where it is needed. The whole process takes fifteen to twenty minutes and should not be drawn out further. A review of the research on Therapeutic Touch, Michael Lerner's *Choices in Healing* (1994) indicates that this can be an effective way of relieving pain, accelerating wound healing, improving the body's basic metabolism, enhancing relaxation, and improving the quality and duration of sleep. It has reduced stress in premature infants and diminished the anxiety of cardiovascular patients.

When the intent is to heal and help by touch, the practitioner enters an I-Thou relationship with the patient, and is herself nourished by the energy she draws from herself by centering. At the Commonweal Cancer Help Program in Bolinas, California, participants with cancer work with each other, so that each person gives and receives healing touch. There is a mutuality, empathy, and bonding that happens in the program. The circle becomes an I-Thou container. Centering is enhanced. Michael Lerner, president of Commonweal, comments that in this context the giving and receiving of simple touch is profoundly positive. "It often induces deep feelings of mental, emotional, and spiritual healing, and sometimes has significant effects on physical symptoms as well."[2]

Life Force and Healing Energy

There seem to be parallels between energy that children need from maternal sources, in order to grow and thrive, and energy that sick people need to heal. When we are sick or little, there is an instinctive need to be mothered, or have mother around. I remember those years when my children were little, when they were very active and growing in size, and relative to the energy it must have taken simultaneously to grow and to remain in perpetual motion, they didn't seem to eat that much. It felt to me as if I were giving them my energy to grow on, just as I'd given them milk when they were newborns. After putting them down to sleep, I had the urge to go to bed also. If I resisted the impulse and stayed up an hour or so longer—enough to generate more of my own energy—I got my second wind.

In order to live, babies need to have more than their physical needs taken care of. Food, blankets, and clean diapers are not enough: Babies in wartime England who were cared for in large impersonal nurseries had these, but were not held, cooed to, and loved, and so often they died of what is now called "anaclitic depression." Love and touch were missing, and newborns died when these essential ingredients were lacking. Neglected toddlers with the diagnosis of "failure to thrive" have managed to survive but at times with their physical and mental growth stunted from a similar deficiency of love and touch. Isolation and loneliness at any age make us susceptible to disease; there is less resistance to illness—from catching a cold to hastening death. Men who are widowed, for example, are at risk of dying during the year following their wives' deaths, especially if their wives were their only source of both intimacy and community.

When we are mourning or ill, the presence and touch of our caregivers

2. Michael Lerner, *Choices in Healing: Integrating the Best of Conventional and Complementary Approaches to Cancer* (Cambridge, Mass.: MIT Press, 1994), p. 365.

nourish us. Touch may actually be life-sustaining, especially during periods when a person is between this world and the next, when whether
they will live or die is in question, and one thing may tip the balance.
Marion Woodman described such a precarious time for her. She was alone
in India and almost died of dysentery. She recalled passing out on the
tile floor of her bathroom. Coming back to consciousness, she described
being out of her body, looking down from the ceiling at her body lying
on the floor, caked in dry vomit and excrement. She returned to her body,
and gradually regained strength and health. When she was able to get
out of bed and out of her room she began going down to sit in the hotel
lobby. There a strange encounter occurred:

> I sat on the end of a couch writing a letter. A large Indian woman in a
> gold-trimmed sari squeezed between me and the side of the couch. Her
> fat arm was soft and warm. I pulled away to make room to write. She
> cuddled against me. I moved again. She moved. I smiled. She smiled.
> She spoke no English. By the time I finished my letter, we were both
> at the other end of the couch, her body snuggling close to mine. Still
> fearful of going outside, I returned to the lounge the next day. The same
> dignified lady appeared; the same game went on. And so for several days.
> Then as I was leaving one morning, an Indian man stepped up.
>
> "You're all right now," he said.
>
> "What do you mean?" I asked, startled at his intimacy.
>
> "You were dying," he said. "You had the aloneness of the dying. I
> sent my wife to sit with you. I knew the warmth of her body would
> bring you back to life. She won't need to come again."
>
> I thanked him. I thanked her. They disappeared through the
> door—two total strangers who intuitively heard my soul when I was
> unable to reach out my arms. Their love brought me back into the
> world.[3]

Marion had not known that an Indian man had sent his wife to sit
next to her, too close to be socially appropriate between strangers, or

3. Marion Woodman, *The Pregnant Virgin: A Process of Psychological Transformation* (Toronto: Inner
City Books, 1985), p. 179.

why, until she recovered and he told her that he had recognized that she was dying and so directed his wife to do this. I think Marion got a transfusion of energy, of life force, of compassion, through direct contact with the Indian woman's body. Her soul had hovered on the ceiling above her sick body, and though she had returned to her body, the Indian man must have seen how tenuous a connection she had to it.

In a lecture at a humanistic medicine conference in Germany, I heard Dr. Jeanne Achterberg describe something similar. When her husband, Frank, had a heart attack, Jeanne climbed into the hospital bed with him in order to give him her vital energy at a time when his life was at risk. Before she left for the hospital, she had mobilized a prayer network as well.

I inadvertently did the same for my mother when we both believed she was dying. Thinking she was about to die, I got into bed with her to hold her and to be there as daughter and midwife at her soul passage. I held her through the night, and in the morning, the risk had passed.

The transfusion of energy from a healthy person to an ill person in order to strengthen them and aid in the process of healing is as acceptable an Eastern concept as expecting positive effects from a blood transfusion is to us in the West. A healthy person is seen as having an abundance of *prana* or *qi* and an ill person a deficit. Anyone who lays on hands intentionally gives or channels energy to a person who is open to receive it.

Powers of Repeated Prayers

There is power and solace in prayers that have been said millions of times. Every religion has some prayers that are recited over and over again. These prayers seem to tap into collective human experience, into the morphic field of our species, into the collective unconscious that both influences us and to which we contribute. When we say these prayers, we draw from this power. There is usually a rhythm to such prayers, and their words have the power of affirmations or mantras; in their repetition and cadence, they shift consciousness, working themselves into the subconscious or unconscious, becoming what we believe.

Reinhold Niebuhr's Serenity Prayer has a special place in Alcoholics Anonymous and in many of the recovery programs that share its principles. It is a prayer that offers direction to those in situations beyond their control, but where it nonetheless matters how we respond, what we do. Whether the life-threatening, life-changing illness is alcoholism, cancer, or some other serious disease, this prayer applies. I know people who say it many times each day and when I think that all of us are spiritual beings on a human path, this prayer seems especially important:

> *God, give us the grace to accept with serenity the things that cannot be changed, courage to change the things which should be changed, and the wisdom to distinguish one from the other.*

Recently, I heard about a man with AIDS, who was on a respirator; he was expected to die but didn't. The prayer he had learned and repeated, over and over, which specifically asks for angelic support, was "The Guardian Angel Prayer." Many adults remember learning this in the first or second grade of Catholic parochial schools. One version is:

> *Angel of God*
> *My guardian dear*
> *To whom God's love*
> *Connects me here.*
> *Ever this day,*
> *Be at my side*
> *To light and guard*
> *To rule and guide.*

Like the Serenity Prayer, it is one that has been said millions of times, and if there are such things as morphic fields that we add to and draw from, saying this one over and over would draw on the same collective experience. To pray is an act that banishes fear and has a direct effect on the body's immune system.

Prayer and I-Thou Links

Soul companions hold each other in consciousness—and commonly, in prayer as well. The importance of being held in consciousness and prayer when we undertake a psychological, physical, and spiritual journey or ordeal is something I know makes a difference, even if there is no way I have of proving it. To ask someone, "Please pray for me," or to be told, "I'll pray for you," is a soul-to-soul communication. To respond and do it is a choice that evokes love. When we know that we are being prayed for, we feel loved. When we pray for someone, it is an act of love. There is something about prayer that taps into a larger source of love, and the person praying and the person prayed for are linked through this love.

There are soul links between people for which prayer is the link itself. Dominique Lapierre, in *Beyond Love,* tells of the founding of a soul link between every sister in Mother Teresa's Missionaries of Charity and a disabled and suffering person, which began with Mother Teresa and Jacqueline de Decker, a Belgian nurse. For two years, prior to meeting Mother Teresa in Calcutta, de Decker had lived alone and worked among the poor in Madras, trying to relieve suffering. During these same two years, Teresa had sought permission to found a new order that would serve the poorest of the poor. In 1948 the two women met, and de Decker committed herself to Teresa's project. She would be Teresa's first companion in the Order of the Missionaries of Charity. However, while she was preparing to follow her friend into the slums of Calcutta, Jacqueline became crippled with spinal pain, possibly related to trauma from a diving accident in adolescence, and had to return to Belgium for care. In Belgium she was operated upon several times, had fifteen grafts, and was in a full-body cast.

Lapierre tells us:

On realizing that she would never be able to return to India to work with her friend, she wrote Teresa a heart-rending letter, the desperate farewell of a woman who saw her dream and the meaning of her life slipping away from her.

Sometime later, she received a blue aerogram bearing the postmark of the central post office in Calcutta. In the space of a few lines, Mother Teresa outlined for her a unique project: the creation of an association that would weave across land and ocean, the links of a mystical communion between those who suffer in their bodies and need to be active, and those who are active and need the prayers of others in order to be so. "Today I am going to propose something to you that will fill you with joy." Teresa wrote to her Belgian friend that October 8, 1952. "Will you become my twin Sister and a true Missionary of Charity, being in body in Belgium but in soul in India? By becoming spiritually linked to our efforts, through the offering of your suffering and your prayers you will share in our work in the slums. The work here is tremendous and needs workers but I also need souls like you to pray and suffer for the success of our undertaking. Will you accept to offer your suffering for your Sisters here in order that they may have the strength each day to carry out their works of mercy?"[4]

Thus was born the Link for the Sick and Suffering Coworkers of Mother Teresa, affiliated to the Missionaries of Charity, which Lapierre described in 1990 as still coordinated by Jacqueline de Decker, despite her age and chronic pain. The first links were formed between twenty-seven severely handicapped and incurably sick people and the first twenty-seven sisters who had gone with Mother Teresa to serve the poorest of the poor in the Calcutta slums. Thirty-five years later, the Link involved thousands of people.

4. Dominique Lapierre, *Beyond Love,* translated from the French by Kathryn Spink (New York: Warner Books, 1991), p. 145.

The Alchemy of Prayer

There is an alchemy of prayer: for the person prayed for to be affected, so must the person who is doing the praying also be changed. To pray for someone can be done as a spiritual service, which is also a spiritual practice, as with Mother Teresa's prayer links. One's own pain and suffering from a chronic condition, which might otherwise be meaningless if we are alone and isolated in pain, become the means through which compassion for the suffering of others and the wish to relieve that suffering is undertaken.

As a personal experiment in transformation of suffering through prayer, a person with a chronic and disabling illness might decide to pray for a particular person. It might be someone in a helping profession he or she would like to support through prayer; it could be someone on the frontlines, making a difference as a social, political, or environmental activist; someone who is helping others in ways that matter to the person who is praying. Or it could be to support another ill sufferer or to sustain the faith and work of someone close to us. The commitment would be to pray for that person two or three times a day for several months. To make such an agreement is to embark on a spiritual journey, to believe that prayer can be a means through which others are helped, and to be faithful to the commitment.

If you believe that praying will make a difference, it will—in ways that are psychological as well as spiritual. In prayer, the ego is in relationship to the Self, to the archetype of meaning within us, as well as to the sacred that surrounds us. It is this encounter and communion that nourishes and replenishes the soul. Maybe angels multiply when we pray, surrounding us and going out to those we pray for. Maybe angels are packets of divine nourishment, care packages needed at a body and soul level.

Prayers for others are expressions of love. With love, the more we give, the more there is and the more we have. The same principle applies to angels, if to pray is to send angels.

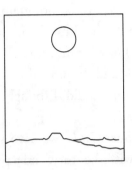

PRESCRIBING IMAGINATION

The *Little Engine That Could* is a healing story.[1] If you take the essence of it as medicine, it will help make you well. It has no side effects and is free, but it requires do-it-yourself effort and the magic of imagination. I am talking about the use of visualization and affirmations in getting well. My left-brain medical colleagues may roll their eyes at this as gullibility, or be incensed at this as nonsense, as they overlook or don't even consider ways to enhance the healing response of the body. Their authority is intimidating, as is their certainty that nothing could be potent unless it is also potentially toxic or invasive. I see this element in allopathic medicine as a "guy thing," with its emphasis on overpowering and conquering disease. Maybe it has to do with being right-brain challenged, and thus lacking a sense of approaching illness from a healing perspective. Visualizations and affirmations assume that there is a mind-body connection, that what you feel and think influence getting well or staying sick.

1. Watty Piper, *The Little Engine That Could* (New York: Platt and Munk 1930).

In this children's book, the little engine pulled a load that was bigger than he had ever attempted over a mountain, by saying to himself, "I think I can, I think I can, I think I can," and then, as he gained momentum and confidence, "I know I can, I know I can, I know I can," until he was over the hump, and coming down the other side, with "I thought I could, I thought I could, I thought I could" to the cheers of children.

In *The Little Engine That Could,* we have a story with an emotional message, pictures to go with the story, and a positive statement that the engine (and the child) says over and over again. Each one of these three elements has something in common with ways people have of mobilizing healing through drawing on physical and psychological resources. Identifying with the story happens emotionally. Without knowing the word *metaphor,* the child uses the story of the little engine as a metaphor: which means she knows that she is not an engine, *and* she knows that it is her story. The child makes a connection between the engine's successful effort to make it over the mountain and the particular difficulty she has to overcome.

The inspirational stories we hear and believe and apply to ourselves get into the marrow of our bones to influence healing and recovery. The cells of the body respond, through peptide receptor sites, to true stories of remarkable recoveries, stories that are metaphors for what the body is capable of doing when we have a positive emotional response to these stories. They are transmitted in ways that we are just learning of—as energy or biochemical reactions—to activate or inspire the healing response.

Visualization

Visualization is a mind-body technique that a child instinctively uses when applying *The Little Engine That Could* to some difficulty in her life. As a technique to heal, to reduce pain, or to mobilize one's immune system, you can learn to create pictures in your mind that are as simple as the illustrations in children's books. When you visualize a metaphor, the physiology of the body responds. Just as the child sees the illustrations of the train when she identifies with the story, so do patients see the story they are telling their bodies through visualization. The ability to activate the archetype of the child, to suspend logic (and skepticism) and enter the magical world of the inner child for whom metaphor *is real* makes visualization work for adults.

Visualization and Cancer

The use of visualization in the treatment of cancer was pioneered by Dr. O. Carl Simonton, a radiation oncologist. In 1978 he coauthored *Getting Well Again*,[2] the book that drew national and international attention to the use of visualization in the treatment of cancer. I became acquainted with him and what he was doing in 1973. At that time, he was fulfilling a military obligation at the medical facility of Travis Air Force Base in northern California, when I heard him lecture and show slides about the connection between visualization and healing at a small Jungian conference in southern California.

Carl was a charismatic, engaging, and persuasive speaker who was convinced that there was not only a connection between the psyche and the development of cancer, which others in psychosomatic medicine had already suggested, but a connection between the mind and the body that could also be mobilized in the successful treatment of cancer. He was using a combination of visualization, meditation, and psychotherapy with the oncology patients who were on his ward for radiation.

His approach made intuitive sense to me, and shortly thereafter I went to observe what he was doing firsthand. I went on the ward, watched him work with a group of patients through a two-way mirror, talked with him about what he was doing, and how he himself was inspired by the results of teaching visualization to one of his first patients.

2. All references to Carl Simonton are taken from O. Carl Simonton, Stephanie Matthews-Simonton, and James L. Creighton, *Getting Well Again: A Step-by-step, Self-help Guide to Overcoming Cancer for Patients and Their Families* (Los Angeles: J. P. Tarcher, 1978; New York: Bantam, 1980).

This was a sixty-one-year-old businessman with advanced throat cancer. He was very weak, his weight had dropped from 130 to 98 pounds, he could barely swallow his own saliva, and he was having difficulty breathing. He had less than a 5 percent chance of living for five more years, which was the benchmark for survival.

Carl wanted to help him, but the man was dying. Being in the hospital and getting treatment was not working, but here was Carl, one of his young doctors, telling him that he could do something besides lie there passively, getting sicker. He had nothing to lose. He listened while this persuasive and positive resident told him about the mind's ability to influence the body, and how the immune system worked to rid the body of cancer. All he would have to do to help himself get better was learn to relax into a meditative state of mind and visualize his cancer, the radiation treatment, and his white cell response, as vividly as he could.

He agreed to take from five to fifteen minutes, three times a day, to do this. He was to compose himself by sitting quietly and concentrating on the muscles of his body, starting with his head and going all the way to his feet, telling each muscle group to relax. Then, in this more relaxed state, he was to picture himself in a pleasant, quiet place—sitting under a tree, by a creek, or anywhere that suited his fancy, so long as it was pleasurable. Following this he was to imagine his cancer in whatever form it seemed to take.

Next, Carl asked him to picture radiation therapy as millions of tiny bullets of energy that were directed at the part of his body that was riddled with cancer. The normal cells in the area would also be affected, but they could withstand the radiation, which would kill the cancer cells. Then he was to see his white blood cells coming in, swarming over the weakened cancer cells, picking them up and carrying them off along with the dead and dying ones, and flushing them out of his body. In his mind's eye, he was able to visualize his cancer decreasing in size and his health returning to normal.

The results were spectacular. The radiation therapy worked exceptionally well; the man showed almost no negative reaction to the radiation on his skin or in the mucous membranes in his mouth and throat. Halfway through treatment he was able to eat again. He gained strength and weight. The cancer progressively disappeared. Two months later, there were no signs of cancer.

The patient was an executive, who was used to giving orders and having them carried out. He heard what Carl had to say and trusted him. That he could tell the white cells in his body to get rid of cancer cells did not take a leap of faith: once Carl said it was possible for him to order them to do what he wanted them to do, he assumed the authority with ease. It was, after all, no different from giving an order and having it executed.

Following the remission of his cancer, the patient decided on his own to use visualization to cure his arthritis, which had troubled him for years. He mentally pictured his white cells smoothing over the joint surfaces of his arms and legs, carrying away any debris, until the surfaces become smooth and glistening. His arthritis symptoms gradually became less, and although they returned from time to time, he was now able to go stream fishing regularly. Then he decided to use visualization to improve his sex life, and got rid of his problem of impotence that he had had for over twenty years. At the time *Getting Well Again* was initially published, six years had gone by and his cancer was still in remission; he was sexually potent and little affected by the arthritis.

As great as the influence visualization and Carl Simonton had on this patient, he in turn had an enormous effect on Simonton. When I talked with Carl about this particular patient, I recalled listening to Dr. J. B. Rhine, the father of parapsychology who made ESP a household expression, speak of the spectacular ESP abilities of his first significant subject. Fate brought an exceptional subject to each man, very early in their careers. While others could doubt and even ridicule them, what they had believed possible was proven *to them,* by an exceptional subject.

Imagination and the Immune System

Visualization supposes that imagination can have an effect on the body at a cellular level. The homely subject of warts contributed to my openness to the connection between the mind and cells. Before children were taken to dermatologists to have warts removed, children and adults prescribed various Tom Sawyer remedies, all of which worked for somebody: it might have been sump water applied during a dark moon, or a string that had been soaked in urine wrapped tightly around the base of it; whatever imagination devised, warts would drop off. Warts are not malignant, but they are tumors, abnormal masses of cells that grow where they don't belong.

Anyone who can relax and meditate can use visualization, by telling a story to the body in pictures and creating a drama for the white cells to enact. The white cells circulate and keep us healthy by reacting to bacteria, viruses, and other infective organisms of all kinds. They also have to do with allergies, with vaccinations, and with resistance to cancer. Immune cells learn to recognize invading organisms, and they specialize.

The white cells might be visualized as good soldiers attacking and destroying invaders. Or inspired by the video game Pac Man, the white cells might be imagined as Pac-men rushing through corridors gobbling up malignant cells, which are black and round. Or, the white cells might be seen as a clean-up crew, a janitorial service that takes away abnormal dead and dying cells that have been weakened or killed by radiation or chemotherapy. Or, the white cells might be seen as bubbles of a foaming cleanser that dissolve the bad cells. These are all tried-and-true imagery.

The most effective images for you are those that feel intuitively right, ones that are tailored, created, or adopted as your own. For example, when war or battlefield scenes were suggested as the metaphor, combat scenes between the immune killer T cells and the cancer cells worked well for *Terminator* or *Rambo* movie fans. It was "too much carnage" for women who rejected this choice of visualization and didn't like this kind of movie, either.

After I mused about prayer as a means of sending healing and protective energy—or angels—to those we pray for, I thought about the medieval theologians who debated about how many angels could dance on the head of a pin, and suddenly I could envision white cells as millions of microscopic guardian angels who protect me by circulating through all the tissues of my body, able to recognize and rid my body of what should not be there. Maybe this image comes close to what really happens: maybe an angel is a quantum of subtle energy that we can influence or direct by our visualizations and prayers to heal or protect us. Maybe they are the messages that activate or energize the immune system of white cells to look after us.

Skeptics can hardly be blamed for not believing that the complex immune system could be directed, much less even affected, by exercises of the imagination. I might have had this same reaction, except for experiences that I had before being introduced to visualization, so that when I heard Simonton describe the use of visualization in the treatment of cancer, and the effect of the mind or emotions on the development of cancer, it not only made sense, it followed logically from what I had already observed about the response of the body to metaphor images.

Visualization and Physiological Changes

In an introductory hypnosis course that I took, we were told to imagine a control room in our head. We were to go into the room and see a control panel with levers on the wall. Each lever controlled the flow of pain sensation to a specific part of the body. It was suggested that if we pulled a lever down, it would cut off sensations of pain from that part of the body, which would become numb—an arm, for instance. To test the result, we stuck pins through that arm, and didn't feel any pain. I learned, on myself, that if a person was in a mild trance state, the body could be directed to do something by imagining a metaphor that tells the body *what* to do.

In that same course, we were told to imagine that one hand was in a bucket of ice water and the other was in a bucket of warm water: as a result, one hand became cooler, the other warmer, with a difference in skin temperature between the two.

Since I had already learned how imagination and physiology went hand in hand, the idea of mobilizing the immune system through visualization made sense to me.

Why Not Try?

In 1984 author Reynolds Price found that he had a large cancer in his spinal cord that was pencil thick, gray, ten inches long, and descended downward from the hair on his neck. It could not be surgically removed. The shape reminded him of an eel. Hearing a tape of Simonton on the use of visualization to harness the body's own powers of self-healing, Price spent hours in the effort to mobilize his immune cells. He even drew colored pictures of "the eel," studied his colored drawings, and then with his eyes closed, visualized white cells swarming over his image of the eel and consuming it. He comments:

> Not that I had great faith in the method. At times I felt that my brain was running some rejected sequence from Disney's *Fantasia,* the war of the good mice against the bad.
>
> At such times I'd come close to sharing the general medical suspicion that alternative therapies amounted to pointless shadowboxing. But surely the practice had to be harmless, no one looked on and laughed at my thoughts, the thoughts took up time which hung on my hands; and in a hard but invisible illness, slack time can be as devastating an enemy as disease itself. All these years later, I'd still commend such visualizations to anyone besieged by renegade cells— whether cancer, resistant tuberculosis, another microbial disease, autoimmune diseases like rheumatoid arthritis and MS, or even AIDS. I wouldn't suggest that the method "works" infallibly or often;

but I suspect it did me some real good, if not in destroying tumor cells, then in its gift of meditative calm, the sense it gave me of an ongoing grip on my mind at least.[3]

Visualization and Reversing Heart Disease

Reversing coronary heart disease is the focus of Dr. Dean Ornish's work. His program of stress reduction techniques, group support, and changes in diet has produced improvements in functioning, prevented heart attacks, and helped reverse already existing heart disease. In *Stress, Diet and Your Heart,* Ornish described the reasoning behind the use of visualization in his program. He too was impressed by the change in temperature in the hands when people visualized putting one hand in ice water and the other in hot water, an effect that comes about through blood vessels that either bring more blood to the hand, which warms it, or constrict flow, which cools the surface temperature. He reasoned that if visualization could enable a person to influence blood flow to the hands, then perhaps it could enable a patient to increase the blood flow to the heart.[4]

In his instructions to patients, Ornish begins with the statement "Your body responds to pictures in your mind," and then step by step, he suggests how to visualize. What to visualize was up to the patient. One man visualized removing the blockages in the coronary arteries with bottle brushes; another used a Roto-Rooter with the same effect. Vaporizing and drilling through blockages were images that two others had.

Some people can have a visualization "prescribed" because it is easily adopted and speaks to the psyche of that person. However, the more you are engaged in the process, the better, it seems to me. Creating the visualization involves you in what the disease is, what the treatment does, and how the healing response of the body can help. Like a graphic artist or a playwright, you are then called upon to translate your disease,

3. Reynolds Price, *A Whole New Life: An Illness and a Healing* (New York: Scribner, 1994), pp. 58–59.
4. Dean Ornish, M.D., *Stress, Diet and Your Heart* (New York: Penguin, 1982), pp. 9, 115–128.

the treatment, and your body's healing response into the language and visual imagery of metaphor and to imagine being well again. Suppose your life depended upon drawing a series of pictures for someone to follow. Imagine that they are the only instructions. Psyche and body have to come together in this, and the authority that accepts a particular metaphor as being right is the inner one. You may find yourself learning that there is an inner knowing and to trust it—which is as significant in following a healing path in your life as it is important in creating an effective visualization.

Affirmations

The Little Engine That Could also demonstrates the use of yet another mind-body technique called affirmations. The little engine (and the child) repeats encouraging words to itself over and over again. The words have the cadence of a drumbeat or a heartbeat: "I think I can, I think I can, I think I can, I think I can." The message is an affirmation, and the repetition of an affirmation in the midst of difficulties can have an effect on the body and the psyche. An affirmation is also a story: it's a story one tells to oneself, about oneself, often *before* it comes true; it is a story that has an influence on shaping the outcome.

Affirmations are repetitive positive statements we make to ourselves. They can be as simple as the Little Engine That Could saying, "I think I can, I think I can, I think I can," instead of focusing on how big the mountain is or how heavy his load, or how difficult his task, or how little he is himself, or how inexperienced, or how he could run out of fuel. Instead of resenting the load or comparing it to others, The Little Engine That Could said, "I think I can, I think I can, I think I can." This is the way of affirmations. They program the current situation positively and assume success.

Repetition literally changes the structure of the brain. In "Issues in Physics, Psychology and Metaphysics: A Conversation," written with psychologist John Welwood, theoretical physicist David Bohm said, "Any thought which is repetitious, strong, full of powerful emotion,

and a sense of absolute certainty . . . will leave 'grooves' in the brain."
He went on to explain, "When experiments have been done with
radioactive tracers to see what happens inside the brain, every idea,
every feeling creates a radical redistribution of blood in the brain. If you
kept on bringing blood into a certain pattern all the time, you would
begin to grow more cells there, and less cells somewhere else. And also,
with very strong thoughts, the synapses would get very fixed."[5]

Affirmations are a conscious effort to program the mind, often as an
antidote to negative statements originally said in anger or fear by parents or other authority figures, then repeated to one's self, or perhaps to
counter one's own pessimism, in an effort at least not to make an "old
groove" deeper. Affirmations need to be said with conviction and feeling and, to be most effective, out loud while facing yourself in a mirror. At the beginning, you are like an actor working on saying a line to
sound convincing. It is a practice and it takes discipline to do. Like
meditation or visualization (or dieting or exercise), affirmations require
a commitment of time and duration to work.

Affirmations and Louise Hay

I became interested in affirmations and why they work after being invited
to be co-keynote speaker with Louise L. Hay at a healing and rejuvena-
tion conference in Tuscany, Italy. In anticipation of meeting her, I read
her books, *You Can Heal Your Life* and *The Power Is Within You*.

I found her own life story one of the most inspirational stories about
overcoming adversity, including cancer, that I can remember. Her
childhood was one of emotional deprivation, poverty, and trauma; she
was raped at five by a neighbor (who was sentenced to prison), yet
blamed for letting it happen, and further abused emotionally, physically,
and sexually. She was a runaway from home and school at fifteen, had
an unwanted pregnancy and a child given up for adoption at sixteen.

Her adult life continued in a similar vein until she went to the

5. David Bohm and John Welwood, "Issues in Physics, Psychology and Metaphysics: A Conversation," *The Journal of Transpersonal Psychology*, vol 12, no. 1 (1980), p. 30.

Church of Religious Science and became absorbed in being a student of metaphysics and healing; three years later she was eligible to become a practitioner, and began working as a church counselor. She entered the ministerial training program after that, and began seeing clients and giving lectures, putting together her first book on metaphysical causations of physical illness. Then she found that she had cancer.

To heal herself, she went into psychotherapy and expressed the bottled-up feelings from all the abuse she had suffered; as she also pieced together why the abusive people in her life had done what they had, understanding and compassion for them grew into forgiveness. She sought help from a nutritionist, cleansed and detoxified her body with a diet that was mainly green vegetables and with a course of colonics. Believing that she had to love and approve of herself to survive cancer, she stood in front of a mirror and said to herself such things as, "Louise, I love you, I really love you," which was very difficult. As she persisted, she found that in situations where she would have berated herself, she didn't. With these mirror exercise affirmations and other work, she was making progress.

Louise's belief was, "If I had the operation to remove the cancerous growth and also cleared the mental pattern that was causing the cancer, then it would not return. If cancer or any other illness returns, I do not believe it is because they did not 'get it all out,' but rather that the patient has made no mental change. He or she just re-creates the same illness, perhaps in a different part of the body."[6] The choices Louise made about what to do, and her commitment to these beliefs, worked. Her cancer disappeared and did not return.

Programming Positive Thought

Like a plane going into a slow tailspin, becoming sick can depress the mind, and then the mind depresses the healing response of the body, and round and round, and down and down, one goes.

Affirmations are a simple means of counteracting the critical and judgmental words that go around and around in the mind, heaping

6. Louise L. Hay, *You Can Heal Your Life* (Carson, Calif.: Hay House, 1984, 1987), p. 220.

blame on you when you are ill and vulnerable, making matters worse by making you feel worse about yourself. It's a deliberate effort to substitute a positive set of words in place of ones that otherwise play over and over, making you feel defeated and afraid.

Just because the idea of affirmations seems so simple, it does not make saying them easy. Deciding that affirmations might help, for example, you might begin with a positive statement, such as: "I deserve good health," or "I am lovable," only to find that it is hard to say. A part of you may think that doing affirmations is ridiculous. Susan, my surgeon friend, confided that when she began she felt sheepish even though there was nobody else there. However, she stuck with it, until she believed what she said. A decade later, if she wakes up feeling anxious or negative about herself, she stands in front of the mirror and says her now "grooved" affirmations to counteract it.

Effective Affirmations

Jan Adrian taught workshops on affirmations before she was diagnosed with breast cancer and then founded "Healing Journeys: Cancer as a Turning Point" conferences. She, like Louise Hay, intuitively recognized that she must do more than get treatment for cancer, that she had to change her mental set. For her to change her life, for cancer to truly be a turning point, she knew that she had to change her grim view that life is a struggle and everything is hard. Knowing that affirmations work but that each word must be carefully chosen, she created this affirmation for herself: "My life is *becoming* easier, more fulfilling, and fun." Like Susan, who had difficulty saying a statement that began "I *am,*" Jan got stuck on saying an affirmation that said "My life *is* . . ." before it was so; however, she could say and believe "My life *is becoming* . . ."

Jan suggests that you take what is the most difficult or most negative thought and construct a sentence that is its opposite, which becomes the affirmation—or prescription. For an affirmation to be potent, Jan emphasized the "three Vs: Verbalize, Visualize, and Vitalize." You say the affirmation aloud—you verbalize what you want to believe. Then see yourself as your affirmation, visualizing yourself or your situation as if it has already happened. Adding the emotion that you would feel if what you affirmed were truly so will, in turn, vitalize you. In her experience, the right affirmation affects the body and psyche: "you can see people light up from inside."

Affirmations turn out to be like telling yourself what you yearned to hear from the people who mattered to you. They become a means toward seeing and cherishing yourself as you should have been by others. You substitute positive, supportive, optimistic words for the ones you would otherwise be telling yourself.

Imagination Comes First

I think of affirmations and visualizations as tapping into the power of the imagination, which is a generator and transformer, a force that precedes and shapes who we become, and what we create and achieve. Whenever we attempt something new or difficult, we have to be able to imagine it before it becomes possible. It's the combination of inspiration and perspiration that brings about tangible results. Healing is no different, especially if you have a life-threatening illness. Here, for example, your doctor's attitude and words are a powerful help or hindrance to your getting well or not.

I think of doctors as having the equivalent of green thumbs or black thumbs in gardening. The doctor who is a healer taps into the power of positive imagination and vice versa. He or she recruits the innate healing power of nature by expectations that come through words and attitude that *this* will help, that *this* will heal, and whatever the medicine does—or the surgery or the radiation—is enhanced by positive expectations. The message is passed on to the body through *emotion-colored pictures* in our mind, and the body responds.

This is also what happens when we use visualizations and affirmations. We produce, write the script, and cast these emotion-colored pictures that enhance the healing process, focusing the energies of mind and body on the possibility of positive results.

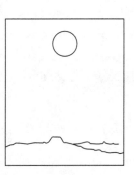

RITUALS: ENACTING MYTH

Rituals mark the major, collectively observed gateways to endings and beginnings: Birthday parties, New Year's Eve and New Year's Day events, christenings, engagements, marriage ceremonies, graduations, retirement parties, and memorial services are such events. In recent years, women who consider the body sacred and honor the physical transitions have begun to celebrate the onset of their daughters' menstruation and their own menopause, which, along with motherhood, are three major biological phases of women's lives. These physical initiations, sometimes called the blood mysteries, change the body and psyche of women; each ushers in the next significant phase of her life.

A life-threatening illness is also a transition and an initiation into a phase of life that is precipitated by changes in the body. With the onset, there are events and crises with physical and spiritual consequences. There are major changes in roles, and there is need for emotional and spiritual sustenance for all concerned—all of which make this medically mandated situation a time when ritual can make a difference to the soul. For example, entering a hospital to undergo a surgical or medical procedure that has life-or-death consequences is a soul event, and rituals that acknowledge this provide psychological and spiritual support that help keep body and soul together through this passage.

An Instinct for Ritual

When an I-Thou element enters a ritual, divinity is present, linking the participants with each other and with the greater mystery. There is a shift away from the trivial into the eternal. Or, described psychologically, there is a shift into the archetypal realm. When ritual space and experience have already been created and practiced, this may happen immediately upon saying an invocation or holding hands or bowing heads or lighting a candle. The wish for some ceremonial acknowledgment of what is happening arises in people at times of crisis, when spiritual help is needed to transform the situation or to face fate. This is when people want to receive the sacraments, or create a ritual for themselves and invite grace or healing to enter.

Significant rituals that are created rather than traditional, depend upon their potential for symbolic meaning and their capacity to touch emotions, to invoke the sacred. To create a personal ritual, intention and contemplation of doing such a thing are the beginning. If it is to be a creative process and a powerful rite, soul tells you what the ritual is for, and whom you want to participate in it. What others have done can serve as the inspiration.

For example: Prior to chemotherapy, Patricia was told that she could expect her hair to fall out, probably in clumps. She had been lent or given some wigs and hats to try on in anticipation (shared like outgrown baby things used to be years before, in what felt like a previous lifetime), which was a practical way of preparing for this. On a whole other symbolic and spiritual level, she had been wanting to call her friends together for a healing ritual. It was then that she heard of women undergoing "chemo" who cut their hair off or shaved their heads instead of waiting for their hair to fall out. They took control of the situation. Some had made it into a ritual event. She had an immediate *Yes!* response to the idea.

Many women instinctively cut their hair when they need to be strong, so to see this as a symbolic empowering ritual was one possibility. A Buddhist friend told her that a shaved head in one of the Buddhist traditions symbolized enlightenment, which also made sense. She heard of one woman who was moved to share a friend's ordeal, and another who was moved by the suffering of others, each of whom decided to cut off beautiful, long hair in a symbolic act. On taking vows, nuns in many traditions shave their heads. It is an act with archetypal significance that is also very personal and individual. For created rituals to touch deeply, there has to be both an archetypal underpinning and a personal element.

Her ritual was simple, solemn, *and* spontaneous fun. She asked her close women friends to come. A sacred space had been created inside the house; a circle of stones had been laid out with a candle in the center, for the circle of women who stood, held hands, and invoked spiritual support for what was to be done. She thanked us for coming, for our love and support, and told us why she had decided to do this. Some of us contributed what we knew about the meaning of having the head shaved, and all of us were awed and uncertain about what to expect.

Once done, she could not change her mind. What would it be like? What would she look like? There was an energy in the circle now; it was indeed a sacred space, and a transformation we were there to witness had already begun in her. Our friend was seated and we were standing, yet she seemed tall—or rather, there was a presence and poise about her that made her seem so. As she related to us later, she felt loved and supported—and elated, liberated, and terrified by what she was doing and what was about to happen.

Patricia asked her adult daughter, who had never done anything like this, to do the cutting. First her hair was shorn with scissors, then it was

cut to a uniform half inch with an electric razor. Her friends were her
mirrors; we reflected what we saw back to her: courage, beauty, and a
head with good bones. With her head shaved, she looked like a baby, a
Buddhist monk, an elf, like Nefertiti—or a new self. There was laughter and relief, it was spiritual and empowering of us all, and it was also
"girls doing hair," commenting, laughing, and supporting our newly
shorn, brave friend. It was a ritual and a party.

Rituals Prior to Surgery

Often having a sense of what others have done strikes a note, and we
intuitively sense what elements are right for us. This has been so for
many women prior to a mastectomy, who have been told by others to
take the time to acknowledge the loss they are about to experience, to
remember pleasures and pain associated with the breast, and the ful-
filled and unfulfilled real and symbolic aspects of their lives that the
breast represents, and to thank the breast for the sacrifice it (or she) is
about to make. If there is an I-Thou relationship between a woman and
her spouse or lover, ritual expression will likely include lovemaking that
focuses on that breast for the last time. Candles, flowers, sage or
incense, champagne, a special place may be elements.

A ritual may take place in the privacy of her bath: a woman can caress
the breast (or the abdomen when it is a hysterectomy that is to be
done), reflect and remember what she has felt and experienced to do
with breast or uterus, be thankful or grieve for what she has experienced
through this organ, or not had as an experience. Lovemaking, childbearing, nursing, pleasure, pain, positive or negative self-image, all that
it has been and anything that it represents may come to mind, and in
silent recollection or in a private dialogue with the part of the body that
will be sacrificed, it is a ritual. Tears and prayers may follow. Hearing
what some women have done in this way may inspire others, men as
well as women, to acknowledge the meaning ritually and to address the
loss consciously, prior to entering the hospital.

Elements of Ritual

Rituals are outer expressions of interior experience. Some are very private, and shared only with an intimate; others involve larger numbers of people: friends, relatives, or kindred spirits gather together to witness, acknowledge and support a significant passage. It is common in grassroots women's support groups, or circles of friends gathered for this specific reason, to come together prior to a hospital admission, or even before then, for the express purpose of helping their friend—and, invariably, ritual arises.

Whatever makes the space itself a sacred space rather than a social one, enhances the sense of ritual. The sound of a bell, a moment of silence, a prayer, listening to a poem or to music are simple ways to begin. Then the purpose of the gathering might be expressed, which can be to aid and support this friend through what is coming, to do whatever might heal or help.

The telling of the story is part of this ritual. If you are the person who is the focus, how much you tell depends upon who is there. When there are children, relatives, and others present who matter to you, but who aren't people you necessarily have bared your soul to, what you say may not be as revealing as to your best friends. A narrative of events that brings you to this particular threshold is part of the telling. It could include symptoms or what you have been told by your doctor about the diagnosis and what to expect. It can be a time and place to acknowledge feelings of grief and anger, or to speak of shame and fear to do with having to undergo this passage. What might you say?

When a group comes together for a ritual, it is different from a support group in form. It is focused upon one person, and a specific event. You may even have expressed your raw feelings about what you are about to undergo to these people, and now as you tell them what is about to happen and what it means to you, it is something that you have dwelt with and thought about. On the verge of going into an unknown and risky experience, you are now drawing upon the love and support of others, and you are calling it up from yourself.

It is important to be able to recall and remember past ordeals and events which you have survived, learned from, and grown through, at this time. What is now being faced can then be placed within the context of your life. You are the protagonist in your story. You are continuing a journey. You are facing a particularly significant passage, and those who love you need to know this, and know what you need from them.

The others who take part in your ritual may be active participants as well as witnesses. They may have something to say to you, or they may give you symbolic objects to accompany you, representing qualities they want you to have. Or you may want them to keep something symbolic, a tie to you while you are making a descent: colored yarn worn around a wrist, or a ribbon worn for you, as people wore yellow ribbons for men who were missing in action or red ribbons to support people with AIDS.

The ritual may end with prayer, with laying on of hands, with a sound or a song, or with words chosen or spontaneously said. Whatever makes it meaningful, whatever brings your personal community together, whatever you want to do, whatever might help, is right, a freeform, from-the-heart ritual.

Metaphor of Journey

Leaving for the hospital for a diagnostic workup, or the operating room for surgery, or your doctor's office to begin chemotherapy, or the radiation center for a radioactive procedure, not knowing what will be encountered, what will be found or how you will respond, can be like setting off on a journey to an unknown place or an encounter with an unknown power. Friend or foe? Usually others can accompany you only so far, and then you are on your own. Even if they are literally beside you and holding your hand, it is you alone who are at risk.

It's hard to know exactly what you will need from others, but if you either know yourself well or have been on this journey before, you may have some definite ideas about what you might want and not want.

This could include prayers, calls, and visits to the hospital; specific or tangible help with children, errands, food; or work-related coverage—any range of things.

When you have a life-threatening illness, or enter a hospital for treatment, part of the preparation is to take responsibility for the possibility that you may not return, or be as able as now to make decisions. Will you leave the important things in order, just in case? Have you a will? Have you made arrangements for your children? Have you signed a durable power of attorney for health care about how much life support you want or don't want? Have you set aside time to speak from your heart with whoever will be responsible, if you no longer can be? These matters and the people you entrust them to deserve I-Thou conversations, which become sacred moments, ritual exchanges—really—to do with entrusting others with the concerns that are close-to-the-bone issues. Trust from you, pledges in return, hope that this will not be necessary, expressions of love and appreciation, a soul-to-soul conversation, prayer together, a symbolic act—how might you express what it is you are doing at a soul level as you take care of these personal and legal matters?

When Inanna set off for the underworld, Ninshubur went with her for part of the way. Inanna gave her explicit directions about what to do if she did not return, and then said, "Go now, Ninshubur—do not forget the words I have commanded you." Ninshubur did not forget, and when Inanna had not returned after three days, she did exactly what Inanna had said to do.

To do what will help because you want to and can, is the essence of an act of friendship in which the giver and recipient benefit. For many strong and independent people, being on the receiving end is hard. Seen in the light of illness as a soul experience, the lesson gained may be to accept help and feel gratitude—which Inanna did. To the one who freely volunteers herself or himself, and then can be counted on to give emotional support or practical help, even when it becomes a sacrifice, the lesson may be to give help and feel grateful that you can. To give and receive is one and the same at the soul level. Acts of love and trust go both ways.

Parallels to Initiation

Surgery has parallels to indigenous initiations. You are taken from your usual surroundings, occupations, and people, and are prepared for an ordeal. Prior to surgery as in many initiatory rituals, fasting is required—all preoperative orders include "NPO," the initials of the Latin words that mean "Nothing through the mouth." In the morning, you are taken into the operating room, which like ceremonial chambers has undergone purification. You are placed on the operating table, draped, and prepared, as if for a sacrifice. Surrounding you are doctors and operating room nurses, who are a special caste of people who wear gowns, masks, and head coverings, and are set apart and have received special training and privileges, like members of a priest class. Under anesthesia, you lose consciousness, enter another world, and are unaware of what is being done that will change you. When the surgery—or the ceremony—is over, you are awakened and are told what happened to you. You have undergone a transformation and are no longer the same.

Following the operation, you go through a recovery period in which a sequence of food—from fluids only to soft and bland food to a regular diet—is prescribed, an order that recapitulates the feeding of infants. Mobility progresses from lying down, to sitting up, to taking the first steps with assistance, to being ambulatory or able to walk by yourself, which is another recapitulation. And then, there is the interest in your bowel and bladder activity, which is also reminiscent of infancy.

The surgical patient enacts a ritual of death and rebirth, an archetypal pattern that is the basis of indigenous initiations, of inductions into secret societies, and religions in which one is born again. In them all, the initiate dies, is reborn, and is for a time an infant member. This similarity and its underlying pattern makes surgery a ritual experience as well as what it actually is. Because this is so, rituals to prepare for the ordeal and to welcome the initiate back, are fitting from the psyche's perspective.

Medical and radiology procedures are usually much less dramatic than surgery, yet the effort to overcome death or bring someone back to health is no less significant, and equally transformative. They are done in an office or even in the hospital, but you come and go. When the potent medicine is swallowed or enters intravenously, the ritual parallel is entering the temple and receiving a sacrament that will change you from within. Here, too, there are risks, for anything that is potent enough to cure you is often toxic enough to harm you as well.

Radiation therapy is done in special rooms that shield others from what you will receive. You are exposed to invisible light or to streams of invisible particles, or might even have radioactive pellets placed inside you that make you too dangerous for others. Many cells in you die, so that you might live.

In Greek mythology, Zeus once made an irrevocable promise to give a mortal woman anything she desired. Tricked by his jealous wife, Hera, Selene asked to see Zeus as Hera could—in his divine form. He became pure energy—like lightning or a nuclear blast: he was heat, light, brilliance. No mortal could survive this. Before Selene died, Zeus saved the fetus she was carrying in her womb by taking it out and sewing it—transplanting it—into his own thigh. In his divine form, Zeus is a personification of unharnessed radiation that can kill.

It reminds me of high-dose radiation (or high-dose chemotherapy) and the removal of stem cells from bone marrow (which are like fetal cells). This is done because the patient has an otherwise terminal disease, and the radiation or chemotherapy is given in such a high dosage that it would be fatal, except for the removal and transplantation of the stem cells back into the patient afterward. The cells save the patient, as did the fetus Zeus removed from Selene, who in a later myth, as the god Dionysus, went into the underworld and brought his mother back to life.

Ritual in the Operating Room

A number of years ago, my friend Anthea entered the hospital for major abdominal surgery to remove a benign tumor that was growing in her colon. It was the kind of tumor that had a strong potential of becoming malignant, and even though the biopsies had not turned up any cancer cells, she was told that it was even possible that they were already present in an unbiopsied portion of the tumor. She called on me to help her negotiate her passage through the Kaiser Permanente medical system, and luck or synchronicity was with us, in that I had unexpectedly just been in contact with a radiologist there, a friend from my internship years. She told me of her good friend who was the best surgeon for this procedure, and as a medical colleague and a friend of a friend, I made an appointment with him for Anthea and accompanied her to see him. I relate these details, because what I would do on the ritual level in the operating room itself could only have been done with his permission; it required that I have credibility and he be receptive, for what I proposed was out of the ordinary and might seem foolish or weird.

Anthea had a strong symbolic sense of what the tumor represented and saw her admission into the hospital for surgery as an enactment of the Inanna myth. The morning of her surgery, an attendant came for her, and she got onto the gurney, and with me following, she was wheeled down the hall, through the elevator doors into the elevator and taken down to the surgery floor and into the preoperative area. There I changed into surgical garb prior to going with her into the operating room. Mindful of the Inanna myth, we saw each of the doors we passed through as another of the gates.

In surgery, she was positioned on the operating table and draped; the anesthesiologist put in an IV, administered an anesthetic, and put in an airway tube; lights were adjusted over where the incision was to be made, and the surgeon and his assistants, now masked, gowned, and gloved, took their positions on either side of the table. Then, the surgeon turned to me and said, "You can do whatever it is you want to do, now."

I told them, "You know what you are here to do medically and surgically. I would like to say something about what this operation means psychologically and spiritually. We are in a ritual space. It is like a temple space or a holy space that has been especially cleansed and prepared. Everyone in this room is garbed in special clothes. The patient has fasted, been purified, and now lies unconscious on what could be an altar, awaiting what will be done here, with life or death perhaps in the balance. A part of her will be taken out and sacrificed, so that she may stay well. For Anthea the tumor represents emotional pain that she has endured since childhood, it is a manifestation of rejection, disappointment, and unexpressed feelings that could become malignant. It is the suffering part of her that has carried her pain. When it is removed and after it has gone to pathology, she wants to take what remains and bury it in the ground, where it can become part of the earth."

And then I suggested that we take a moment to ask for a blessing upon the surgeon and the instruments. There followed a moment of absolute, palpable silence in the OR, and then without a word, the surgeon picked up a scalpel, and made the initial incision.

Quite possibly, in a religiously founded hospital, a moment of silent prayer or spoken prayer might be routinely said. But this was not my experience. For me it meant crossing over a line. As a medical student and intern, I scrubbed and held retractors. The surgeons were usually autocrats in the operating rooms; some were known to swear and throw instruments on the floor if a nurse mistakenly handed them the wrong one.

It is easier to bring prayer and meditation into the operating room, when you are the patient. Before you are put to sleep, you can say that you need everyone to be silent for a moment for a prayer. This has been done by others. You might ask to do this beforehand or insist on it. Even surgeons welcome divine help, and having the OR full of angels—if to pray is to summon angels—is a comfort.

Post-Surgery Rituals of Transformation

The tumor was removed before it had progressed into malignancy. Anthea did get what remained of what had been excised from her colon (even if it seemed a most peculiar request), and in a private ritual moment, she buried it in the garden of her family home. Her tumor symbolized or concretized negativity, unacceptability, and rejection of deep parts of herself that she had experienced from her family and internalized.

Her ritual followed the example of a childless woman who had had a hysterectomy while she was still in her childbearing years. The loss of a uterus that has never carried a child removes the possibility and dream of ever being a biological mother. For the soul, there is a need to mourn that loss. A ritual done with friends is a way of expressing the loss that contributes to healing it. Anthea's friend obtained her uterus after the hysterectomy. With a ritual involving the caring participation of close friends, she buried it (and the possibility of having a child) and planted a tree over the site of the burial, so that as it became part of the earth, its molecules would in turn become part of the tree; dead tissue that was once her uterus would be transformed into new life. The ritual marked an end and a hoped-for new beginning.

These posthospitalization rituals were symbolic acts meant to invoke change in the person; the intention was transformation of pain and loss into new life. Rituals such as these are symbolic enactments or dramatizations of loss as a part of ongoing life. To ritualize loss is to tap into the realm of dreams and myths, which mark transitions in the language of death and rebirth, where burial is a precursor to renewal, resurrection, or the promise that in time, spring will return. As part of a healing process for the soul, burying the actual tissue that was removed is not necessary—for some people it may make the ritual more significant; for others even the idea is distasteful. Instead, an object that symbolizes the loss is chosen or made, and it is held and imbued with personal significance and meaning.

In the symbolic layer of the collective unconscious, the ways that humans from the beginning of time have marked the end of life as a transition into the otherworld become metaphor for endings and beginnings. Metaphor evokes images and archetypal meaning, which rituals tap into. To consign a symbol into the earth, into the sea, into the fire, or to leave it to the elements in the branches of a tree, are easily incorporated into personal rituals because they are not made up but come up out of the soul.

A nurse-therapist who had had surgery and chemotherapy for breast cancer the previous year came to San Salvador Island in the Bahamas to a women's workshop I was leading. She came with the intention of doing a ritual. She had heard me speak of what my friend Anthea had done, and had come to do something similar. There was a long expanse of empty, private beach, with indigenous scrub growth above it. In the circle preceding, she told of the cancer in the context of her life, what she had been through since the diagnosis, and of her intention to leave her cancer and what it represented to her behind. She thought that she would give it ritually to the sea. Then, as we gathered with her on the beach, she had a moment of deep truth, which made her cry. She couldn't do it yet. She could not bring herself to take what she had brought and physically cast it into the ocean. This was the truth of it. What she had thought she would do came up against unexpected deeper feelings: A *No!* made itself felt. Her mind had planned something that her soul knew was premature. Significant ritual and deep truth go together. Ritual is not a made-up, let's-pretend game to play. It truly does engage us, body and soul.

At such times, it is a matter of asking questions of the soul, until what is right for this particular person emerges. I asked her if she needed to return home with what she had brought with her. A clear "No!" was the response. Answers to further questions revealed that it was a matter of time. At some point in the past, she had wanted to die, and the cancer seemed to be an expression of this. Now, she was moving toward an affirmation of life, and she was making changes in her life, but she was not quite ready to embrace life and give up being a

patient. Ritually what was right—inner gnosis, right—for her, was burial several feet deep, at the waterline. There, below the surface and in
the dark, sand and water and time would work upon its dissolution;
gradually and inevitably it would be transformed. When the proposed
ritual act conformed to what her psyche knew was true for her, she
could go ahead. The small ceremonial burial she performed for herself,
with us participating as witnesses, was intense and powerful, and above
all, meaningful.

Chemotherapy as Ritual

Ritual makes real what is really going on. The trip may look like a routine visit to the oncologist's office, but when you are going to the oncologist's office to receive chemotherapy—especially the first time—it
is not an ordinary event. A patient receiving chemotherapy intravenously may look just like any other patient attached to an IV, but
such is not the case. It can be treated as if it is routine, by everybody;
but to do so is to leave out the soul, to be in denial psychologically, and
not to tap into the powerful healing potential of a psycho-spiritual-
immunological system.

Healing is a subjective response, not merely a physiological one.
Emotions play a significant part in affecting the endocrine system,
which in turn affects the immune system: fear and serenity are subjective states with vastly different physiology.

When I went with Patricia and her daughter Ginna to the oncologist's office for her first chemotherapy, numerous friends were alerted
and were praying for her. She was in a state of anticipation and anxiety,
as the IV was put in and attached to a normal saline drip. Once the line
was in, and the nurse left us, a simple ritual centered her and supported
what was about to happen. Our hands linked the three of us in a small
circle. She closed her eyes and took slow deep breaths, and we in turn
did also, synchronizing our breathing with hers. I led a silent prayer,
and then said something about the healing energy and love that could

flow through our hands to her, and how we were this moment receiving and directing to her the love and support and prayers of all those who cared about her. I watched her face become peaceful; her breathing was naturally slow now and easy. It felt as if we had invited support into the room.

When the nurse returned, the atmosphere had shifted. Patricia was ready to receive chemotherapy in a receptive and meditative state. The most potent of the chemicals was a beautiful red color; the other was an opalescent champagne color. They were given in sequence, with an interval between them. I suggested that she see the red as potent and powerful molecules moving swiftly to those places in her body where the cancer was, that the other cells of her body needed to lie low and be peaceful as the red molecules went by, attracted, like iron to a magnet, to the malignant cells. I reminded her that red is her favorite color, and as a color symbolizes life blood, vitality, passion, intensity, and warmth. In between, she received an antiemetic that prevented nausea and vomiting. Then the second drug, diluted in an IV drip, was begun. This time, she was to see and to direct opalescent molecules to her cancer. These were crystal clear, shining molecules that would poison the cancer cells, which would weaken and die, so that she would live. These medications would help her, they were on her side.

Her son came in at this point, listened, and participated; now there were four of us, so our circle expanded, with him at the foot of the bed. The initial small circle had created a sacred space, and the walls of the room were now its boundaries. Each of us supported her through touch and heart. The nurse became part of what we were doing by her attitude of respect. The ritual space was maintained as she went about checking the IV flow, explaining what was going in, answering questions that we had. There was also small talk and laughter. Once created and felt, a soul space does not have to be somber.

If you go alone for chemotherapy, even with the lack of privacy, it is always possible to create a healing space by closing your eyes, centering yourself by breathing and bringing peace into your body. You create a sanctuary around you by bringing such an image and feeling into your mind and soul. You might see yourself in a healing circle, surrounded by people who love you but could not come with you. Or you might visualize yourself in another setting that is beautiful and comforting, out in nature or anywhere else. You might bring an object that has meaning for you, to hold in your hand. You might repeat something to yourself, or go through a visualization that you have prepared. And always, you can pray.

These ritual ways invite the psyche to participate in the healing of the body by physiological and spiritual means. The same ritual attitude and creation of a sanctuary space can be brought to the bedside if you are receiving a blood transfusion, or the medication is a powerful antibiotic or a steroid. It can accompany oral medication. Whatever is taken medically can be more effective in the absence of fear and when mind and psyche focus upon what it is the medication will do.

The Magic of Ritual Words

Ritual can take a place in a moment, as when two people meet on a path in the Himalayas, put their hands together in the universal prayer position, bow and say *"Namaste";* or, when a Catholic enters church, genuflects, and with the words "In the name of Father, Son, and Holy Spirit" makes the sign of the cross. Ritual shifts us momentarily or for a longer duration out of ordinary mind, into sacred time. Words are part of ritual. Familiar words associated with ritual or religion have power; they may have only been half attended to before, but now in the midst of a crisis, they carry great meaning. The soul listens.

The Twenty-third Psalm read aloud to my dying father had such power: " . . . though I walk through the valley of the shadow of death." It was read to him in our kitchen several months before his death, by his youngest brother Daniel, who is a minister, during that liminal time when there was nothing more that could be done medically, and it was a matter of time before he died:

The Lord is my shepherd, I shall not want;
he makes me lie down in green pastures.
He leads me beside still waters;
he restores my soul.
He leads me in paths of righteousness
for his name's sake.

Even though I walk through the valley of the shadow of death,
I fear no evil;
for thou art with me;
thy rod and thy staff,
they comfort me.

Thou preparest a table before me
in the presence of my enemies;
thou anointest my head with oil,
my cup overflows.
Surely goodness and mercy shall
follow me
all the days of my life;
and I shall dwell in the house of
the Lord
for ever.[1]

When Anthea entered the hospital for her surgery, she had the descent of Inanna in her mind—as a myth she was enacting metaphorically. She had been a cofounder of a women's spirituality organization and had often been called upon to lead rituals for others. Now she transformed her own hospital and surgical experience through ritual, only part of which I am describing. Step by step, or gate by gate, she wove her personal story into Inanna's story, and symbolic meaning into the hospitalization.

She asked one of her friends to accompany her to the hospital to participate in a ritual before entering through the doors—or through the first

1. *The Holy Bible,* Revised Standard Version (New York: Thomas Nelson & Sons, 1953), p. 576.

gate. Anthea had worn necklaces and symbolic clothes that she removed as her friend read "The Descent of Inanna, II: The First Gate," from *Truth or Dare,* by Starhawk. Here is a portion of this much longer poem:[2]

Your great achievements
all the things you do
to prove your value
the emblems of your position
mean nothing down here
They all drop away,
clatter to the ground
The snake rubs her belly on them
Her skin splits
She sloughs it
sliding free
It lies in a heap like an old rag
She has shed
as you have shed
The gate opens . . .

Starhawk's Inanna poems provided a powerful text for Anthea's hospitalization. The next poem began with the words, *"The Second Gate is fear."* Every patient passes through this gate.

Fear doesn't go away
but you walk toward fear
naked
And the gate opens

As I waited with Anthea in her hospital room the morning of surgery, it was my turn to read. This Inanna poem emphasized the need

2. Starhawk, *Truth or Dare: Encounters with Power, Authority, and Mystery* (San Francisco: Harper & Row, 1987), pp. 115–116.

to breathe deep and call, to find your voice, to make noise: *"To pass this gate / you must sing."* Then the attendant came with the gurney, assisted Anthea onto it, and with me walking beside her, she was wheeled down the corridor and through the elevator doors. The pre-op medications and lack of fluids had made Anthea's mouth very dry, which meant if anyone was going to sing, it would have to be me.

The elevator was empty. There was only the attendant and my friend on the gurney, which was fortunate for me (after years of medical training, I felt in my element in the hospital as a doctor; but to perform ritual for the first time in a hospital was something else again). The song that came to mind was a verse from the civil rights song, "We Shall Overcome." I had recently watched a documentary on the Public Broadcasting System. The part that brought tears to my eyes was an incident in Mississippi, during which this particular verse was sung. One night, when people were meeting in the basement of a church as part of the effort to register voters, most or all of them black, they heard the sound of cars pulling up outside the church. Then they heard loud voices of white men and barking dogs, and the lights in the church went out. They were now in the dark, terrified of what was going to happen next. One person began to sing, and then all joined in and sang, *"We are not afraid, we are not afraid, we are not afraid today. Oh deep in my heart, I do believe, we are not afraid today."* As they raised their voices and sang this verse, over and over, the song became true. Their fear dissipated, and as if in response, a miracle happened. The men got back in their cars and drove away. And so I sang these same words, *"We are not afraid . . ."* as we got on the elevator, and the doors closed.

This particular song, like the Twenty-third Psalm, moves us when we hear it or sing it, especially when circumstances are such that we are in a time of crisis and transition. These are affirmations of what we believe and want to be so. They draw upon memory and past meaning, and have power in themselves to move us emotionally and spiritually. Perhaps the explanation is that they tap into archetypes, or evoke a morphogenic resonance. For whatever reason, rituals are enhanced when such music or words are used.

Everyday, Ordinary Life Rituals

Then there are the simple, reassuring acts that people do with one another that are rituals. When two I-Thou companions are separated physically, one in the hospital or rehabilitation center, the other at home, it's the good-night phone call as the last communication at the end of the day, and the good-morning call, first thing. Familiar words of love that end the call, of mattering to each other, of being connected, are ritual words. For rituals are about belonging, and being in a situation that is meaningful; they place us in a context and provide spiritual sustenance as we go through a difficult passage or affirm commitments to be with each other "in sickness and in health." Nighttime rituals between I-Thou couples are extensions of childhood bedtime rituals, which are also I-Thou moments in which the child feels beloved, is given assurance of being loved, and is left to sleep safely through the night.

Sacrifice or Scapegoat

Rituals are also a means of reexperiencing a major event in a symbolic way after the fact. Rituals can help us mourn or celebrate changes that have already happened, or acknowledge the completion of a passage. Rituals then become part of the process of letting go of the past and going on. With this in mind, I brought pounds of clay with me to a retreat and workshop I was leading for women who were recovering from cancer. The clay was available to women to make a representation or a symbol of the part of the body that had been removed or treated for cancer, which might then be used in a personal ritual.

As the clay is shaped, memories, thoughts, and feelings come to the surface; sometimes hands seem to mold the clay unconsciously, and only when it is finished does the mind know what it represents. When women set out to make a representation of the breast or uterus that was removed in surgery, feelings toward the organ itself often arise, or an inner dialogue takes place as if between the woman and the organ, which is revealing. Feelings of apology or gratitude may arise. Some find that they deprecated, neglected, or even hated this part of their bodies. Especially when the surgery was done for cancer, what often arises spontaneously is the archetypal meaning of sacrifice: *This part of me was sacrificed so that the rest of me can live.*

This surgically removed part of the body might also have functioned symbolically as the scapegoat. In ancient rituals the scapegoat was the sacrificial animal upon which people placed their fears, sins, or whatever the community wanted to rid itself of; when it was banished, it took away the negativity that was ascribed to it.

When a breast or uterus is removed, feelings about reproduction, sexuality, sensuality, and one's sense of womanhood came to the surface. The meaning and mourning of a removed uterus is affected by the woman's joy or pain about pregnancy, childbirth, abortion. Feelings about the loss of a breast depend upon whether it was a beloved or neglected part of the woman, cherished or denigrated by her or by her husband or lover; whether it was a source of sensual pleasure for herself and another; whether she wanted to nurse a child at her breast and now will not, or whether she had breast-fed her baby. It is not just the part of her that is removed, but the part it played or can no longer play in her life.

Metaphors can serve as guides to meaning. Is there a symbolic correlation between the sacrificed part of your body and your psyche? To muse metaphorically is to look at events in waking life as if they were dreams: What does this symbolize? What is the metaphor or analogy? If I had a dream in which this part of me were diseased or removed, what could it represent? If loss of this part of me was the price I paid for something, what was it? If this part of me was sacrificed so I might live, what will I do with my life now? What would recovery mean? How might this illness be a significant chapter in my life story? What meaning can I make of what is happening to me now?

Seeking answers to such questions requires that we go within, because the answers are there. In each of us there is a need to live our own story, not someone else's expectations or assumptions of who we are. Often life-threatening illnesses provide the impetus to find a lost thread of meaning, which is our personal myth and our soul's reason to be here. What did we come to do? What did we come to learn? Who did we come to love? What did we come to heal?

Answers to Soul Questions

Meditation and ritual are related; prayers are often part of rituals, and rituals take us into meditative states of mind. It is in being meditative that answers to soul questions come. I think of this receptivity as a state of quiet and stillness; it's like waiting for the stirred-up waters of a pond to settle until it becomes mirror smooth and clear, and what lies below can now be seen; or like being on the edge of a clearing in the woods and realizing that if I quiet myself and am receptive, that shy rabbit or deer that I caught a glimpse of out of the corner of my eye might come closer. Gnosis, feelings, intuitions, insights, images, memories, and the thread of meaning that connects us to them are the wild and precious, instinctual revelations of our own nature that come to us, when we seek answers to soul questions in meditation. *The soul will reveal itself as nature does* when we turn inward, still our minds, and wait.

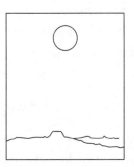

12

HELPING EACH OTHER

I don't remember exactly when it dawned on me that nothing in my life goes to waste, that *anything* that has ever affected me deeply might someday be an empathic connection to what someone is telling me. It was more than an insight; it meant that there was meaning in my own suffering, that anything that I have lived through might some-day be redeemed if it enables me to help someone else. At first, I could see it applied to those of us who do psychotherapy, then I realized that it applied to people who transform suffering into creative work—into poetry, art, drama, or fiction, drawing the essence from their own lives. Then I could see that this could be true for everyone—anyone who was able to see both the uniqueness of his or her own suffering and the uni-versality of suffering, grows in compassionate understanding, which is reflected in their actions and relationships with others. Soul has a growth spurt when we feel for ourselves and others, and *do* something.

People who either deny their own suffering, or narcissistically feel that they alone suffer, can't empathize with others who suffer. This fail-ing limits their development.

At a soul level, compassion leads to helping others, to creative work that expresses and taps into emotional depth, and to community. To care for others as you would want them to care for you, and to love one another, grows naturally out of compassion.

Compassion as the Turning Point

I believe that people who survive a life-threatening illness, which becomes a turning point in their lives, have come through a transformative soul experience as well as a physical crisis. There may have been a complete recovery, or a remission of indeterminable length or shortness, after which priorities are changed. The result is a growth in creativity or service as expressions of compassion and shared humanity, or a new appreciation and involvement with family and friends. I see how gratitude and serving others are linked to the soul and how love for others, for one's self, and for life becomes connected when a life-threatening illness is a turning point for the soul.

Survivors who are grateful for life and health often have a deep sense of having been spared for something. "God still has something for me to do" is how many people who have survived close calls or are surviving put it. This sense of having something yet to do, or knowing what it is, has to do with soul. In Jungian psychological terms, it has to do with *individuation* because it grows out of who we are and what we have learned from experience, from our joys and sorrows. An individuation path is personal and unique. At the same time, every individuation path is an archetypal journey, which means that the underlying shape of such an undertaking is a human pattern. It has to do with a universal longing to do what we came for.

A Life of Significant Soil

When we emerge from a descent through the valley of the shadow of death, and recover from the ordeal of such an illness, the body has survived. The soul questions come next: What will grow out of this experience? How will this change my life? What purpose might it serve? How may it contribute to having a *life of significant soil*?[1]

Sometimes a phrase from a poem captures a spiritual essence for me, such as "The life of significant soil" from T. S. Eliot's *Four Quartets*. For one measure of a life is what grows out of it. Having a life of significant soil means being both the soil and the organic gardener. We become fertile soil when the seeds within us develop and grow, when we "compost" past experience, dig deeply, and attend to this piece of earth that is ourselves. Life has meaning when we birth and tend to new life that comes out of our bodies or minds or souls, develop talents, support and matter to others, and appreciate what we have. This is a life of significant soil.

Erik Erickson, the psychologist who provided us a developmental understanding of the stages of life, described the issues of the middle adult years as generativity versus stagnation. Thinking metaphorically as I do, the question is: a life of significant soil versus a wasteland? There is no new life, no fluidity, nothing green or juicy growing in a wasteland. This is lifeless and depressed psychological soil, the emotional and spiritual landscape where diseases of the spirit often begin as addictions and then progress to illness.

Reunion with Persephone as a Return of Health

After her daughter Persephone was abducted into the underworld by Hades, and all her efforts had failed, the goddess Demeter sat in her temple, depressed. As goddess of grain, she was the most generous of the goddesses, the maternal archetype, who could affect the fertility of the earth. Now, Demeter no longer cared if the whole earth died. Nothing grew. There were no green shoots, no blossoms, no new life anywhere. Earth was turning into a wasteland.

Nothing would grow unless Persephone was returned to Demeter, and as famine threatened to eliminate the human race, Zeus became

1. T. S. Eliot, "The Dry Salvages," in *Four Quartets,* p. 45, line 233.

concerned that if this occurred, there would be no one to worship him. So he sent Hermes to bring Persephone back.

Demeter was in her temple grieving when she heard the sound of a chariot outside. We can imagine how she felt when she realized that it was Hermes bringing Persephone back. She rushed out of her temple and ran toward her daughter, as Persephone, who never thought she would ever see her mother again, leaped out of the chariot. When Persephone's feet touched the barren earth, flowers and green grass sprang up under her. Spring had returned.

The return of the divine child is metaphorically what ends a depression or a descent into the underworld of illness. Joy, innocence, youth come back into the psyche. Spring is the return of health, of growth of creativity.

When gratitude accompanies the return of health and vitality and there is compassion for others who still suffer, a deep desire to help others can grow out of the experience. When this is so and a means of service is found, a generative life or a life of significant soil results.

Illness as a Life-Altering Passage

When an illness is truly a turning point, it is not merely a return to what was before, but a life-altering passage. It can be an extraordinary shift, such as Albert Schweitzer's was. In his early forties, Schweitzer became ill, his health and future uncertain. After two operations, he recovered completely. Not only was his health restored, he had been transformed spiritually and psychologically, and now wanted to alleviate the suffering of others. As a result, he established a hospital and cared for native Africans, who would otherwise have been without medical care. Schweitzer wrote of his illness as an initiation into "The Fellowship of Those Who Bear the Mark of Pain":

> Those who have learned by experience what physical pain and bodily anguish mean, belong together all the world over; they are united

by a secret bond. One and all they know the horrors of suffering to which man can be exposed, and one and all they know the longing to be free from pain. He who has been delivered from pain must not think he is now free again, and at liberty to take life up just as it was before, entirely forgetful of the past. He is now a "man whose eyes are open" with regard to pain and anguish, and he must help to overcome those two enemies (so far as human power can control them) and to bring to others the deliverance which he has himself enjoyed. The man who, with a doctor's help, has been pulled through a severe illness must aid in providing a helper such as he had himself, for those who otherwise could not have one. He who has been saved by an operation from death or torturing pain, must do his part to make it possible for the kindly anesthetic and the helpful knife to begin their work, where death and torturing pain still rule unhindered. The mother who owes it to medical aid that her child still belongs to her, and not to the cold earth, must help, so that the poor mother who has never seen a doctor may be spared what she has been spared. Where a man's death agony might have been terrible, but could fortunately be made tolerable by a doctor's skill, those who stood around his deathbed must help, that others, too, may enjoy that same consolation when they lose their dear ones.[2]

Norman Cousins describes how he came across this same passage and had a burst of recognition. Cousins, as a boy of ten, had been sent to a public sanatorium for tuberculosis. "The pain I felt was not one of sickness but of loneliness. It was the pain of being detached from everything warm and meaningful and joyous in life."

After Cousins recovered, he described: "Even after I was able to accept fully the fact that I could live a normal life, I carried with me the feeling that I had the obligation somehow to pay back. The sense of debt was much more than an intellectual one. It lay deep in my bones,

2. Albert Schweitzer, *On the Edge of the Primeval Forest.* From *Albert Schweitzer: An Anthology,* ed. Charles R. Joy (Boston: Beacon Press, 1947), pp. 287–88.

and I had no way of ignoring it. Indeed, from the moment I walked out of the sanatorium and looked back at my Sunday perch on the old wall near the entrance, I knew that my life would be unbearable unless I could find some way of making good a debt I couldn't quite define but that I knew would be with me as long as I lived."[3]

Xerox copies about Schweitzer's "Fellowship of Those Who Bear the Mark of Pain" were given to me by Beth, a psychiatrist whose membership in this fellowship was earned through a psychiatric hospitalization. There are no surgical scars or calcifications that show up on X-rays of the lungs to mark old, healed tuberculosis; emotional wounding was the source of her pain. She had begun medical school, when emotions and confusion that she had bottled up through years of abuse and isolation in childhood and adolescence could no longer be contained. Drawing on an inner wisdom to know what she needed, she admitted herself to a locked psychiatric ward, where the chaos and self-destructiveness within her could be safely contained. Following this experience, she was able to return to medical school and then go on into a psychiatric residency. She became a skilled and exceptionally sensitive psychiatrist with a deep sense of service. She is especially drawn to working with difficult and disturbed patients, whose acting out, self-destructiveness, and symptoms are related to childhood abuse. These are mostly women who look psychotic, but whose illnesses are expressions of traumatic stress syndromes—like the psychological casualties of war.

Compassion in the Midst of Suffering

It's not just after recovery but in the midst of suffering that affiliation with the suffering of others can grow. When people stay in a hospital for a length of time, the particular ward or wing or floor with its corridors, waiting areas, nursing stations, supply rooms, and hospital rooms becomes a small village populated by patients, regular visitors, and staff. During my father's hospitalizations for cancer, the faces of other visitors

3. Norman Cousins, *Albert Schweitzer's Mission* (New York: W. W. Norton, 1985) pp. 130, 133.

became familiar, and something of the travails of other patients was known. When a friend "became ambulatory" after surgery, and I accompanied her on her prescribed walk, the journey was like walking up and down the sidewalks of a village. At first, she was hooked up to an IV bottle, which hung from an apparatus with wheels that she held on to like a staff. People we passed nodded, smiled, and often said something encouraging.

The longer a hospitalization, the greater the sense of community. Concern and compassion for others can grow in the midst of your own difficulties. If the life-threatening illness leads to the possibility of suicide, a psychiatric ward becomes the village. Each new admission and discharge changes the population. Relationships form on all psychiatric wards; patients grow to know one another, especially if there are therapeutic community or group process meetings.

Fate shared with others in the hospital may be the first expansion of soul. Beyond this is compassion for all others who similarly suffer, of which Schweitzer writes. And beyond this is compassion for all sentient beings who share the planet with us. It is the transpersonal element—the inner, spiritual experience of connectedness to a greater whole—that is truly transformative.

Transformation of Ereshkigal

Author Stephen Levine, known for his work with dying people and grief work with survivors, tells of his experience with a woman who was hospitalized with bone metastasis, cancer that had infiltrated the bone and caused her agonizing pain. In her suffering, she was an embodiment of Ereshkigal, who greeted Inanna with such hatred that she was struck dead. If looks could kill, this patient would have murdered many times over:

> Her lifestyle and her way of relating to the world were such that she had mercilessly judged all those with whom she had come in contact. She had been a tough businesswoman and a difficult parent—to such

a degree that, although she was apparently dying of cancer, her children would not visit her, having been pushed out of her heart and out of her life so often.

This woman had never met her grandchildren. Each nurse, doctor, or visitor who came into her room was greeted with anger and profanity. So she was usually alone in her misery, wrapped in self-pity and blaming others for her torment.

She was a picture of suffering Ereshkigal, alone and groaning, "Oh, oh, oh, my insides."

Then, Levine described the transpersonal experience that she had, which can be seen as a profound initiation into Schweitzer's "Fellowship of Those Who Bear the Mark of Pain." One night, after six weeks in the hospital, she was in excruciating pain, and instead of resisting, she drew a breath into it and something in her shifted:

> She surrendered for a moment and allowed the suffering to move through her, not resisting it as though it came from outside or was another's fault, but giving herself to it as her own. She said later that in that moment—when the turbulent waters of her lifelong resistance and suffering broke through and swept over her as she lay on her side with enormous pain in her back, hips and legs—she experienced herself not as that woman in the hospital, but as an Eskimo woman dying in childbirth. A moment later, she said, she was a black-skinned Biafran woman nursing a starving child from a slack breast, dying of hunger and disease. The next moment, she was another woman, lying beside a river in that same fetal position, her back crushed by a rockfall, dying alone. Image after image arose, which she described afterward as feeling the suffering of "ten thousand people in pain."

The transformation that grew out of this moment was remarkable. The experience opened her heart to the suffering of others as her own, and her own pain as a connection to others. Levine described her as having become a totally different woman:

> In the next six weeks, until she died, her room became the center of healing within the hospital. Many of the nurses spent their breaks there because it was the place where love was most radiant and evident. Within a week, after she had asked her children for forgiveness and pleaded for their return to her life, the grandchildren she had never met before were sitting next to her on the bed, playing "with Grandma . . . with Grandma's sweet, soft hands."
>
> During those six weeks, the pain in her body diminished and the pain in her mind began to dissolve as her heart opened to encompass more and more life, more and more of that which is alive, and to touch the pain of all sentient beings with mercy and loving-kindness. We witnessed in that room one of the most remarkable healings we had ever seen. Although her body continued to deteriorate and she continued to be drawn gradually toward death, she died as healed as anyone we have ever seen.[4]

Her healing was obviously not physical, it was a tremendous inner shift that healed her spiritually and emotionally. Compassion was the healing force that broke through her isolation and opened her heart to others. It healed the separation, the illusion that she was alone. I have the impression that this woman's experience is far from unique, even though the particular images that she had were uniquely her own. Many other people have had similar transcendent moments occur in the midst of great pain, which led to compassion for the suffering of others and the desire to help.

My own occurred toward the end of labor, when waves of deep pain went through me with each longer and longer contraction. At some point, I intuitively knew that what I was experiencing was pain that

4. Stephen Levine, "The Healing for Which We Took Birth," in *Healers on Healing*, ed. Richard Carlson and Benjamin Shield (Los Angeles: J. P. Tarcher, 1989), pp. 198–99.

women from the beginning of time have known, that I was no different, for all of my education and accomplishments, than any of them. Along with the pain that flooded through me in waves, came a new affiliation, a connection with all women, that was my initiation into the women's movement.

Dissolving the Shell Around One's Soul and Heart

Stephen Levine's account of this woman and her transformation also reminded me of Ebenezer Scrooge in Charles Dickens's *A Christmas Carol.* He was a stingy, mean-spirited, and miserly rich man; "Scrooge" is an archetypal figure inside many resentment-filled, bitter people of any age. He had no bonds of affection with anyone, was too cynical to celebrate Christmas, and looked upon Bob Cratchit and Tiny Tim's holiday spirit as stupid and out of touch with reality. When the Ghost of Christmas Past took him back through time to see himself as he was as a younger man, he saw people he once loved who loved him, reconnected with feelings he once had, and witnessed the alienating choices he made. He *felt* remorse for the past, which enabled him to open his heart and be touched by the simple joys and warmth of Bob Cratchit's family. He was thus aghast when the Ghost of Christmas Future showed him what was to happen to them. He was ready to do anything in his power to keep Tiny Tim from dying, and keep sorrow away from this family. When he realized that it was not too late for him to make changes to protect them, he was relieved and grateful. At the end of the story, a warm and happy Scrooge shared Christmas with the Cratchits.

Scrooge lives inside people who cannot feel love for others or from others. When "Scrooge" forms a hard shell around the soul, it is the hard nut that needs to be cracked, in order to reveal the innate qualities of innocence, vulnerability, trust, connection to others, lovability, and readiness to love, which we all come into the world with as newborn souls.

When there is a shell around a person's soul and heart that needs to break open or dissolve, it will be through expression of emotions and feeling that often begins with grief. Grief from loss, disappointments, betrayals, from traumas of all kinds, that moves like a force of nature through the body, wells up with tears and sobs that come from such depths that one marvels where it had been stored. One is bare-souled, newborn, open to feel for others and for one's self, as a result. An inner witness to the grief comes into consciousness as an interior presence, an observing self who feels compassion for one's own suffering and for others who suffer. When soul and personality join together, what one does and who one is become coherent and integrated. Feelings, words, and actions come together. When a life-threatening illness brings about such a transformation and the psyche and the body are healed, work as an expression of compassionate action is often an ingredient in the new life and may even be an element in the recovery itself.

Scrooge became compassionate, as mythical Ereshkigal and Stephen Levine's patient also did—when the walls of bitterness and isolation that separated them from others dissolved. Compassion begets compassion: compassion toward others begins with the ability to feel our own hurts, remorse, sorrows, and griefs. Until it is safe to have feelings, they are held in and held back. In families where tears are ridiculed and the model is denial of pain, to reach feelings takes an initiation into them in adulthood. In environments where compassion and safety are norms, this happens. For men in the men's movement that began with the writing of poet Robert Bly, author of *Iron John,* this happened in gatherings where men reached in and back to their early years, and could express what they found there, which was grief about their distant, abusive, or nonexistent relationships with their fathers.

Sometimes, it is a life-threatening illness, our own or that of a loved one, that begins this process of feeling our own feelings instead of being numb to them. When the floodgates of emotion open, a compassion for others, a sense of shared humanity, of community, often follows.

Helping Others, Healing Ourselves

Lawrence LeShan emphasized that in order for cancer to be a turning point, the physical, psychological, and spiritual aspects of the person must be treated in order to restore and maintain health. In the area of spiritual growth, he said, "I do not regard a patient as finished until he or she is spending some time and energy in work demonstrating concern for more of the human race than the self and immediate family. I have former patients working in the Big Brothers, Big Sisters, ecology and peace organizations, in the Fortune Society and many other similar areas." One of his patients commented that " 'It feeds a part of me I never knew was there.'"[5] The motivation and choice of work needs to grow out feelings of compassion and concern for others and the satisfaction of doing so. The impetus is a spiritual one.

Caryle Hirshberg and Marc Ian Barasch quote Madame Guo Ling, the founder of the Cancer Patients' Recovery Club, a social support network with 40,000 members in China. She maintains that *giving back to society is an integral part of recovery.* Her organization, like Albert Schweitzer's hospital in Africa, grew out of her own suffering and recovery. She had been diagnosed with a terminal gynecological malignancy, underwent several unsuccessful surgeries, and then was sent home to die. Her remarkable recovery involved adapting and practicing an ancient martial art, visualization, and movement of vital energy; now known as Guo Ling Chi Gong.[6]

Another example of this same motivation toward service is Elaine Nussbaum, who told her story in *Recovery: From Cancer to Health Through Macrobiotics.* She wrote, "I know that I want to give back, to reach out to others, to teach, to encourage, to inspire, and to offer hope to those who may be suffering. I want to help people, to spare them the anguish and the agonies that I suffered, to share the experi-

5. Lawrence LeShan, *Cancer as a Turning Point: A Handbook for People with Cancer, Their Families, and Health Professionals,* rev. ed. (New York: Plume, 1994) pp. 134–135, 140.
6. Caryle Hirshberg and Marc Ian Barasch, *Remarkable Recovery* (New York: Riverhead Books, 1995), p. 23.

ence of a macrobiotic recovery, to offer an alternative to degenerative disease."[7]

Nussbaum began by writing her book. After her recovery from disseminated uterine sarcoma that had metastasized to her spine and lungs, she went back to school and received a master's degree in nutrition. She has been a nutritional consultant for the past decade. Though the pain and suffering that she and her family went through are in the past, I'm sure that she draws upon what she experienced when she counsels others. Obviously, she is a living example for others that it is possible to recover. The work she does now would not be possible had she not made a descent into pain and terminal cancer, and returned.

Compassionate Action

In October 1989 I was one of seven psychiatrists and psychologists (the others were Daniel Goleman, Stephen Levine, Daniel Brown, Jack Engler, Margaret Brenman-Gibson, Joanna Macy) who engaged in three days of dialogue with His Holiness, the Fourteenth Dalai Lama, who received the Nobel Peace Prize that very same week. He is considered an incarnation or manifestation of the divinity of compassion, and a bodhisattva—a soul who has achieved enlightenment in a previous life and has voluntarily reincarnated to help others. To be actively in service to others is the heart of a bodhisattva spiritual practice. These discussions furthered my thoughts on the experience of suffering and the nature of compassion as inseparable from involvement.

I asked him, "Is it enough simply to be compassionate, or must we act with compassion?" He replied, "It is not enough to be compassionate. You must act. . . . When there is something that needs to be done in the world to rectify the wrongs with a motivation of compassion, if one is really concerned with benefiting others, it is not enough simply

7. Elaine Nussbaum, *Recovery: From Cancer to Health Through Macrobiotics* (Tokyo: Japan Publications, 1986; distributed in U.S. by Kodansha International through Harper & Row), pp. 207–208.

to be compassionate. There is no direct benefit in that. With compassion, one needs to be engaged, involved."[8]

Further along in the dialogue, Daniel Brown mentioned the results of social psychology research on altruistic action, in which many people in situations where they could be of help to others do not get involved and simply ignore the situation, and those who do, act from outrage rather than from love. He pointed out that survivors of childhood sexual abuse *who get healed* from this, react with outrage and become involved.

Outrage and compassion can go hand in hand. Social activists often are outraged at violations of decency and principles and have compassion for victims. Their style may not bear that much resemblance to the Dalai Lama's, but if motivated by a love of principle or of people, animals, or nature, there is an essential similarity. The opposite of compassion is indifference.

The desire to relieve others of suffering is a common attribute among the members of "The Fellowship of Those Who Bear the Mark of Pain," which Albert Schweitzer described. Many vocations grow out of the desire to relieve others of suffering. They are not restricted to the medical or other helping professions, nor do they necessarily require a change in occupation or profession, though this can result. Once anyone wants to help people by preventing or relieving suffering, there are opportunities everywhere. The helping professions do attract people who want to help others, often because they witnessed suffering in their families, and were grateful or impressed or determined to be in a position to do something.

The retired person who becomes a volunteer may find his or her true vocation only then. A volunteer may have a paying job or a career, and know that volunteer work is the true soul-satisfying work. A businessman may become involved in community work and make it possible for employees to take time to do so also. Doing work that is satisfying

---

8. His Holiness the Dalai Lama et al., *Worlds in Harmony: Dialogues in Compassionate Action* (Berkeley, Calif.: Parallax Press, 1992), p. 96.

to the soul has to do with respect and affection for coworkers, feeling that you are making use of yourself and your talents, and doing some good where you are.

Helping others makes us happy. It's one of the secrets of life.

Seeds of Experience

After Demeter and Persephone were reunited, Demeter asked, "Did you eat anything in the underworld?" If she had not, it would be as if nothing had happened. She would be as she was before, a maiden and a mother's daughter, and could resume spending her days gathering flowers. But Persephone had eaten pomegranate seeds in the underworld, which meant that she must periodically return to the underworld.

Metaphorically, eating the seeds meant that Persephone could "take in" or integrate the experience. It meant that she would now go between the upperworld and the underworld—never again as a victim, but as a guide for others. To integrate an experience of suffering is an act of consciousness. It means feeling what happened instead of being emotionally numb and trying to forget it. This is a first step—toward shifting from being a victim of others or a victim of circumstance. An abduction into the underworld can then be viewed as a beginning, a seed experience that grows into compassion for others and the desire to serve them.

The person who recovers or has a remission has been to the underworld and returned. Whether that underworld was a physical violation like rape or incest or an addiction like alcohol or a life-threatening illness like cancer or AIDS, that person now knows about a particular kind of suffering. Then, whether in recovery or in remission, to heed the desire to help others is to redeem the suffering, to transform pain into compassionate action, into service. When this is the case, your suffering was not "for nothing"; it helped you to find your way into work or relationships that engage your soul.

That helping others is also the way to stay on the spiritual path yourself is built into Alcoholics Anonymous and all of the recovery groups that follow the same inspired model. An alcoholic becomes a sponsor for others. A psychiatric patient becomes a perceptive therapist. A cancer survivor tells her own story and is a role model of hope for others. An artist, writer, or poet transforms the underworld experience into creative work. To transform the experience of suffering in these ways is the path of the wounded healer or wounded artist or wounded teacher, who transforms personal suffering into helping or teaching or creativity.

13

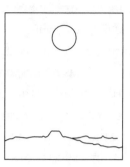

MUSINGS

I wonder what might happen next?" is something I found myself
saying over and over again, when for a time, nothing was pre-
dictable, everything that could go wrong seemed to happen, and
surprises kept turning up. This was on a trip to Greece and the Greek
Islands. To begin with, the size of the boat was too small for the size of
the group, so the accommodations were not adequate. The barometer
fluctuated from frequent weather changes. Twice we literally had to settle on any nearby port in a storm, and each time I heard myself say, "I
wonder what might happen next?" This was a journey that had started
out with an itinerary of what we would do and where we would be each
day, which had to be given up when "circumstances beyond control"
became the theme. With each unexpected thing, some wonderful,
some awful, I would say, "I wonder what might happen next?" For
many days, we called it "the journey from hell," and then there was a
turning point, a few unhappy members of the group left, and there was
a literal sea change; the waters of the Aegean became smooth and a
beautiful blue, and we could frolic like dolphins in it. Basking in the

warm sun that I did not take for granted, I heard myself say once again, "I wonder what might happen next?" Then there was a brilliant sunset on Santorini, an exquisite moment when I said, "Life couldn't be better than this!" The very next day, we averted a near-disaster, and "I wonder what might happen next?" was my response.

Although the trip lasted a little less than three weeks, I learned to wonder "what might happen next?" and carried it over to the whole of my life. I no longer assume that I am in control or that people or events are supposed to live up to my expectations. Instead, I expect that life will be even more unpredictable than the weather. If you muse on this and think back on your life, could you really have anticipated what has happened so far? Weren't there major surprises?

Predicting when a natural disaster will happen or how severe it will be is in the realm of speculation, similar also to the susceptibilities we have to the diseases that could kill us. I live in an area where earthquakes and fires are the dramatic risks, droughts the lesser problem. In other parts of the world, people are at risk for other natural disasters—tornadoes, volcanoes, hurricanes, severe droughts, and floods. Wherever we live—in a particular location or in a particular body—there are susceptibilities to particular natural disasters or particular life-threatening illnesses. There are areas where the risks are greater, and individuals for whom the dangers are greater.

If a life-threatening illness is affecting you right now, I believe that having a "wonder what might happen next?" attitude is realistic, regardless of what you have and what you have been told. A prognosis is only an expectation, much like an itinerary that can never take everything into consideration. A prognosis is like a weather report, which utilizes the most technically advanced instruments and collected data. The doctor, like the meteorologist, predicts and sometimes uses statistics: there is a 90 percent chance of survival, or a 50 percent, or only a 10 percent, for example, is in my mind, about as accurate or inaccurate as predicting rain or the year in which a natural disaster will occur, with one major difference: maybe you can influence the outcome.

If you believe that you are in the percentage who can and will, or could, survive, and do all you can to make it so, it may prolong your life. As long as you are still here, there could be a treatment breakthrough in medicine, or there may be one for you. Or you might get into a delicate balance of power with the illness that is supposed to kill you, when your ability to resist it keeps the disease from progressing. Or you may discover a good reason for living, which you didn't have before, and this may make the difference.

Why Me?

"Why me?" This is the question that often arises when any personal disaster strikes. A life-threatening illness invites the question. Sometimes an answer that places responsibility for the illness on the patient is an acceptable answer for that person, but only if the patient arrives at this conclusion and is empowered by it, as in *If I brought it upon myself by my actions, I can also do something about it.* But in the main, this is a wholly unsatisfactory answer—simplistic, blaming, and twice victimizing the person, who suffers the illness and the blame for it.

Even if you know that you contributed to the situation and blame yourself, whatever you did cannot be the whole cause of it, because others who did the same thing—whatever it may have been—got away with it. AIDS, cancer, traumatic physical injuries, heart disease, all the life-threatening and life-altering illnesses that humans are susceptible to afflict some and spare others. There are times when the margin of error is very great. There are other times when there is no slack whatsoever, and all it takes is one minor infection or one delayed reaction, or one mistake for a life to be at risk.

Job, that good and upright man in the Old Testament who lost health, family, friends, finances, and standing in the community, did not get a satisfactory answer from God to this "Why me?" question.

The wisest and oldest souls among us, however, are probably those who do not even think in such terms, and thus do not ask, Why me?

Reynolds Price, for example, wrote in *A Whole New Life:* "Some vital impulse spared my needing to reiterate the world's most frequent and pointless question in the face of disaster—*Why? Why me?* I never asked it; the only answer is of course, *Why not?* And a lifetime's exposure to the rocky luck of my large family had inoculated me against the need to make an equally frequent claim—that my fate was unfair or unjust. Aware of the troubles of so many likable kinsmen around me in childhood and youth, I'd almost never expected fairness."[1]

When suffering is a universal experience and we know it, we neither assume prosperity, work, love, or health as our due, nor do we rail against adversity, misfortune, or ill health as violations of some agreement that such things should not happen *to us.* Suffering, in one form or another, does go with the territory that is human experience. It is unpredictable in the form it will take, in the intensity and duration, and is not equitably distributed.

Unfulfilled expectations that nothing bad should happen lead to "Why me?" or to "Somebody has to pay for this!" Rage and anger can then take center stage, as a response to illness or disability—or depression results, when these feelings are turned against the self.

When you have a wide and wise perspective on the human condition, as Reynolds Price had, by knowing of the troubles of others, anger at what has befallen you can seem as inappropriate as raging at bad weather, when the response could be to focus on repairing the damage or buttressing against it. Price comments: "Even now I remain puzzled by those occasional friends and counselors who repeated one of the dumber TV-remedies of the time and urged me to let my *anger* out, to bellow my *rage.* Rage at whom or what, I couldn't guess. At a mindless cell proliferating in response to its haywire nature? At destiny and the whole design of my life, if it had a design?"

Manufacturing rage because someone else thinks you should be angry when you aren't or being stuck in self-pitying anger get the

---

1. All references to Reynolds Price are taken from Reynolds Price, *A Whole New Life: An Illness and a Healing* (New York: Scribner, 1994).

patient nowhere. Contrast this with the sort of authentic anger that mobilizes effort, that is an assertion that you matter or that someone else, on whose behalf you are angry, matters; or with an empowering anger enabling one to act decisively and do what needs to be done; anger that is an expression of vitality and of having expectations that you can change something that needs to be changed. This is the anger that Inanna women who integrate aspects of Ereshkigal are able to express. It's an energy that makes it possible to become an exceptional patient, a survivor who is able to get angry if it is called for, if it is needed to get something done right.

Must It Be Someone's Fault?

In blaming and shaming families and cultures when troubles happen, a destructive version of the childhood game of tag begins. Someone has to be "It." For the patient, cruel words remembered from childhood, such as "You brought it on yourself" or "You had it coming," often echo sadistically through corridors of our own minds. Or blame may be couched in words such as "We create our own reality," or explanations such as "Bad karma from past lives," statements which—when only superficially understood and seen through the lens of blame—are New Age versions of "You brought it on yourself" and "You had it coming."

A patient is then weighed down by the same burdens as a rape victim, becoming a carrier of the projections of others who ascribe reasons why this illness happened to this person.

Blame-the-victim "reasons" are punitive. They are very different from objective cause-and-effect reasons, the seeking of which can lead to solutions, cures, and preventive treatment for medical and social problems.

When people are afraid that what has happened to someone else could happen to them, they often distance themselves from the victim. If they can blame the victim, they feel safer or superior, which is the unconscious motivation. Blame is also a way of shifting guilt onto someone else.

It's not just the patients but their families (and their physicians) who can feel responsible and therefore guilty, or blame someone else. When things don't go right, when decisions turn out in hindsight to have been the wrong ones, blame and guilt arise, or at the very least there are the "if only" feelings of remorse or responsibility.

I think, for example, of the "if onlys" to do with my father's cancer, which began with some white patches in the inside of his mouth. My mother was concerned that it was leukoplakia, which can be a precursor to cancer, so she made an appointment for him with an oral pathologist and went with him for the appointment. The pathologist examined him and was absolutely sure that it wasn't leukoplakia. He said that it had the classical appearance of another white, harmless, and often psychogenic condition, and that since my father was a spouse of a physician, he would spare him a biopsy.

When cancer did develop, my mother blamed herself for not insisting on the biopsy. I think my father probably blamed himself for smoking, which he did not do much of and never did around me or even any of his middle-aged siblings, probably because it had been considered a sin in his fundamentalist Christian family. Then there was my contribution to the situation. When the pathologist said that what my father had could be psychogenic or stress-related, I knew that I was the major stress. He had made it clear that he opposed my plans to marry a medical school classmate. I thought he was being unreasonable, and had let him know that I thought so, and would go ahead with or without his approval. I wondered, had I not been such a rebellious daughter, would my parents have accepted a psychogenic diagnosis so readily?

Getting caught up in the "if onlys" cannot change what happens, it can only *contaminate the experience of loss and mourning with blame.* Maybe the situation wasn't even what we assumed: perhaps the oral pathologist was quite correct; when he saw it, it may have been nothing.

Holding the Opposites

One of the earliest deaths from AIDS was a gifted young Jewish poet whose perspective on the shortness of his life was a source of solace for my friends David and Michael, almost two decades later. This was before most physicians knew what AIDS was. During his illness, he was often outraged at the difficulties and obstacles to getting good medical treatment, and at the misdiagnosis and mistreatment that he experienced. Yet, when it was his time to die, he was not angry. He told his friends that there was an old Jewish story that explained why.

"There is a great book," he said, "in which our names are written before we are even born. After each name, there are only two dates—the day we are to be born and the day we are to die."

David, who died of AIDS, found solace in this story when he became HIV+, as did Michael, after David's death. David undoubtedly extended his life, by doing everything he could to combat AIDS and the particular opportunistic infections that came his way. He used his medical training to get information and evaluate every new treatment, and went after whatever was promising.

In Jungian psychology, David was *holding the opposites*—his response to AIDS was not an either/or proposition, not a matter of being either an activist or a do-nothing fatalist. He made decisions as if how long he lived and how well was up to him, and at the same time he believed that when he died was beyond his control. When he found he was HIV+, he knew that he probably would get AIDS, and that once he had AIDS, he probably would die from it, and that did not keep him from putting both off for a longer time than usual, through what he did.

Earthquakes—Real Ones and Metaphors

"The ground gives way under us" was a metaphor I used to describe the emotional impact of an unexpected life-threatening illness. Shock waves move out from an epicenter in an earthquake, and when it is a large quake in a populated area, some people die and others survive. There is a sparing of some and the death of others in a real earthquake, as there are when it is a metaphor for a particular disease of epidemic proportions. Why some and not others? Not as a lament, but as the question that can never be adequately answered.

Several years ago, the San Francisco Bay Area was struck by an earthquake on the first day of the World Series. A portion of an elevated freeway collapsed, killing some people and injuring others. One of my patients and his wife had driven home from the Oakland airport and passed through safely, a scant ten minutes before it collapsed. They had been pleased when their luggage was among the very first to come down the chute onto the baggage carousel. Later, they realized that this stroke of baggage good fortune may have made the ten-minute difference.

People in a University of California Medical Center van were not so fortunate. They were there when that section of freeway collapsed, and there were deaths and injuries among the passengers. This van was one of two that regularly left the San Francisco campus for the East Bay at the same time. On that particular run, a physician got into one of the vans and happened to see another physician, with whom he wanted to confer, boarding the second van. So he left the van he had been seated in and joined his colleague.

Upon crossing the Bay Bridge, the vans would customarily have made a Berkeley stop first and then gone on to Oakland. They would have gone directly on to Oakland *only if* there was no one in that particular van going to Berkeley. On this fated run, the van the physician had left headed straight for Oakland, and was thus where it was when the earthquake struck and the elevated freeway collapsed. The physician lived in Berkeley. If he had not left that van to sit with his colleague, it would have gone to Berkeley first, and there would have been no deaths.

I heard the story because he was telling it to others, and the story was passed on. His part in what happened troubled him, as well it might. And yet, what to make of it? In natural disasters and wars, some people are completely spared and unaffected, some have close calls and know it, some may have no idea how close they were to a disaster, and some are injured, become disabled, or die—as it is with most life-threatening illnesses in ordinary life.

When I fell asleep at the wheel of my car on my way to my own birthday dinner, and missed hitting a telephone pole at fifty or sixty miles an hour by several feet, it felt like my guardian angels had been looking after me. It was a metaphor and a synchronicity: I had once more received the gift of life on my birthday.

A year later, Barbara St. Andrews, an Episcopalian priest who had just turned in the manuscript of a book—writing that I had urged her to do, and been a mentor for—died instead of being spared, probably also by a matter of several feet. She was on her way to a lunch with friends when the car she was driving went off the road and through a chain-link fence. It had metal supports, one of which had to enter the automobile at just such an angle, for it to have killed her.

This time the unanswerable question "Why me?" was about being spared. Why me, and not Barbara?

Two stories made an impression on me when I was in my late teens. I have not gone back to reread them since, not even now as I recollect them—because what I remember is "the story" or message that I got from each of them, not necessarily what was written. One was *The Bridge of San Luis Rey.* It told about a suspension bridge that collapsed, carrying the handful of people who were walking on it at that moment to their deaths. In retracing events that brought each of them to this fate, it became clear that this was not a random, senseless event for any of them. I didn't know the word *synchronicity* then, but I intuitively felt the power and mystery of such a happening, as this fictional event was.

Another was a story by John O'Hara. In it, there was a man who was told that Death was coming for him, and in an attempt to escape this fate, he was hastily preparing to leave for Samarra—some exotic place that left a sound such as this in my mind. Meanwhile Death sees him and, puzzled, remarks to himself, how strange it is to see this man here in this town, when he has an appointment to meet him later, in Samarra.

These stories are variations on the theme that there is a time and even perhaps a place for each of us to die. Maybe each of us has a designated life span, a time to be born and a time to die, that is predetermined; or maybe within certain limits, there is considerable leeway. I think that what we know, believe, and do, does influence our health and can even determine whether we will recover from a disease that could kill us. At the same time, these stories also ring true.

I have come to my own personal conclusion that the timing is not what matters. What we do between being born and dying, is what matters. The point, it seems to me, is to live a meaningful life, however long or short it may be. If a life-threatening illness or a chronic disabling illness is what the soul encounters, then this is the current shape of the soul journey.

When It's My Time, I Want to Be Conscious

There are midlife transitions and late-life transitions and then the last transition that will take us through the veil, or through the mists, or across the river to the other side, or down the tunnel to the light. I hope that I can die well—whatever that may mean—when the time comes. Dying is what we all will do, one day. The second half of life points toward this end, and though we can deny or anticipate it, ready or not, the time will come.

When I was pregnant and knew I would be going into labor and delivery for the first time, I also hoped I could do it well. I did not really know what it would be like, even though I had delivered over one hundred babies and thought I knew what to expect. I found that there was a vast difference between being the doctor in attendance, and being the pregnant woman in labor. Being the woman through whom the baby is emerging is very different from being at the receiving end, helping the baby out—as different as having a first orgasm is from reading about them. I suspect that when I am the person who is doing the dying, this experience, too, will be vastly different from witnessing others die or hearing about it.

Just as I wanted a natural childbirth because I wanted to be conscious, so do I want to be conscious at the moment of my death. Some people want to be asleep when they die, just as many women want to be unconscious when they deliver babies. Also, I wanted my newborns to come when they were ready to come, just as I hope to die when I am ready to go.

When I was present at the moment of my father's death and saw his face infused with joy a mini-second before he left his body, the moment was a gift. Over the years since, others have told me similar stories of the deep peace and serenity they witnessed and felt being with people *whose deaths came when they were ready to go,* even when pain or problems played such an awful part in the last period of life. And over and over again, I hear stories of how the room or the house was filled with invisible yet almost palpable presences, as if others were there to welcome and accompany the soul home from a journey.

A life-threatening illness of any kind and at any age is a psychological and spiritual crisis. If we are lucky and heed the soul message and then recover from the illness, this can turn out to be a physical initiation into a midlife passage. Midlife soul-searching arises when we have lived long enough to know how fast our life has gone by, and something in us says that it matters what we are doing with it. "This is it." This is *my* life, not a prelude to it or a dress rehearsal for it. *Now* is all we have for sure.

Life-Threatening Illness as a Test

Louise Hay, whose books on affirmations I talked about earlier, is an example of a person who already was on a recovery path and already had changed her life, when she developed cancer. She had been a high school dropout, who discovered that she had an intellect and a love of learning. She had begun teaching what she had learned, finding she had a talent and a love for this work. And then she developed cancer. She had taken a major turn for the better, and then it was all tested. Cancer challenged her to commit herself more, to walk her talk—to apply what she taught to her life, which she did.

I have seen this happen to myself and others who already were on a soul path and were doing work based upon beliefs. I found myself, for example, needing to make hard choices which called upon me to follow my own words or not, from *Goddesses in Everywoman*.

Life seems to come along and test us on the principles we stand for and are teaching. It's as if life says, "Let's see if you *really* mean what you say." An ordeal of faith, in which we and our beliefs and relationships must be tested, follows.

Life is very hard for patients with illnesses that have a pattern of progression, or have an acute phase followed by a slow recovery, or have exacerbations and remissions. When the descent means one loss after another, and the list of what you can't do anymore grows, and it's no longer clear how much health will return, it is hard to keep on keeping on. Given the magnitude of this loss, grief and mourning for our former health, for what we once took for granted, is natural and appropriate. And yet, doctors commonly respond to the patient's tears by prescribing antidepressants, or simply by becoming irritated or judgmental.

Sobbing grief is part of the mourning process. Mourning is part of healing and is the soul's reaction to loss, an archetypal experience through which the heart of the mourning individual grows in understanding, and further opens to the suffering of others. Whether you mourn your own lost health or mourn the loss of a beloved, you grieve for what is lost, and come to know more fully than you knew before, just how precious health and life are.

Return of Persephone Accompanied by Hecate

At the end of the myth, when Persephone returned from the under-world, she was accompanied by Hecate, the goddess of the crossroads, whose time was twilight. Hecate was the wise woman and crone who comforted Demeter when she returned from her unsuccessful search for Persephone and advised her to seek the truth of what had happened. It was Hecate who accompanied Demeter to talk with the god of the sun, who had seen it all.

We learn from the Homeric Hymn to Demeter that from the time Persephone returns from the underworld, Hecate *precedes and follows*[2] her wherever she goes. A cryptic notion, physically impossible for Hecate in an embodied form, but possible if she was an invisible spiritual presence or a symbol of the transformation that can accompany a return from the underworld.

As goddess of the crossroads, Hecate could see three ways at once. She could see where we were coming from as we came to the crossroads, and she could see where each of the two roads would take us. I envision her as ancient and wise to the ways or paths that we can take in life, in death, and in between. I think about her as a crone with knowledge of the past and future, and recognize that this makes her a personification of the feared and persecuted image of the witch, whose precursors were the Fates.

Whenever we make a descent and return, if we integrate the experi-ence and now know more about our own depths and how suffering takes us down into the underworld of shared human experience, we gain more of Hecate's particular wisdom. It is body-soul knowledge about cycles of life-death-life. Hecate is the archetype of the midwife, the crone who helps deliver babies or bring new life into the world, and who as midwife at the time of death, helps the soul make a transition. Her acceptance of birth and death and suffering as integral parts of human experience helps us have perspective.

2. References to Persephone's return are taken from "Demeter (1)" from *The Homeric Hymns*, trans-lated by Charles Boer (Irving, Tex.: Spring Publications, 1979), pp. 129, 133.

Each time we make a cycle of descent and return, we gain some Hecate wisdom that we can draw on when another cycle takes us down again, or when we accompany others on their descents. It is no wonder that Hecate would accompany Persephone from the moment she returned from the underworld, and would precede and follow her from that day forward. Persephone could become queen of the underworld and guide for others, because she had the wisdom of Hecate with her.

In the dimly lit recesses of collective memory and mythology, Hecate and her sister figures reside as the Fates, or Norns, or Wyrrd (Weird) Sisters. Crone figures are linked with Fate or Destiny, who weave threads and cut them. Acceptance of Fate comes with knowing Hecate as an inner figure. Words that echo this wisdom are often the only ones that offer comfort to those who mourn—especially when a thread was cut and death came early.

Eleusinian Mysteries

Once Persephone was returned to her, Demeter gave humankind her "beautiful mysteries, which are impossible to transgress, or to pry into, or to divulge." These were the Eleusinian Mysteries, which for more than two thousand years before Christ, was the mystical religion whose initiates did not fear death.

Demeter knew suffering, experienced loss, raged, isolated herself, became depressed, felt powerless and betrayed, and mourned. Like members of Albert Schweitzer's "Fellowship of Those Who Bear the Mark of Pain," once free from pain and anguish, she did not take life up just as it was before, but instead helped those who still did fear death and suffered.

The Eleusinian Mysteries overlapped with Christianity, continuing into the fourth century A.D. Even though thousands of people were initiates, none revealed what the mysteries were. Given the nature of people and secrets, if it were a secret that could be told, it would have been. But if it was a mystical experience—an inner *gnosis*—there would be nothing to tell.

In the past four to five thousand years, first through the Eleusinian Mysteries and then through Christianity, the message that death is not the end has been the same. Only the gender of divinity changed. The triple goddess as Maiden, Mother, and Crone was personified as Persephone, Demeter, and Hecate in the Eleusinian mysteries. It is the Trinity of Father, Son, and Holy Spirit in Christianity.

In one, it was the divine daughter, in the other, it was the divine son who returned from the realm of death. One was abducted by Hades; the other was crucified and placed in a tomb. Each went into the underworld and returned. They overcame death, and in doing so were transformed. The maiden became queen and guide to the underworld. The son became Christ. Return, rebirth, or resurrection then became possible for us, who in some mystical way, could share this same experience.

In the collective unconscious of humankind, as in these two major mystical religions, death is not the end. While the waking ego may be apprehensive at one's own impending death, the dreaming psyche often is not. The dream themes often are of travel, of going on, as if there are expectations of continuity. Then as now, there are ways people know that death is not to be feared—through a near-death experience or faith or an inner source of wisdom, or from being present at a sacred moment, when a soul leaves this world.

The Search for Meaning

> *These are only hints and guesses,*
> *Hints followed by guesses; and the rest*
> *Is prayer, observance, discipline, thought and action.*[3]

Insights from myth, dreams, and intuitions, from glimpses of an invisible reality, and from perennial human wisdom provide us with *hints and guesses* about the meaning of life and what we are here for.

3. T. S. Eliot, "The Dry Salvages," in *Four Quartets* (New York: Harcourt Brace Jovanovich, 1943), p. 44.

Prayer, observance, discipline, thought, and action are the means through which we grow and find meaning.

A life-threatening illness brings suffering and soul into our lives. It brings us close to the bone as it strips us of nonessentials and insignificant concerns. It makes us aware of how short life is and how precious good moments are, and connects us to others and to the suffering that only compassionate acts can alleviate. If it does not kill us, it indeed makes us strong.

Times of crisis are opportunities for accelerated lessons in what it is to be human. Assuming that we are spiritual beings on a human path, rather than human beings who may be on a spiritual path, then the most difficult times in our lives also teach us and test us and often pull us back onto a soul track or a heart path—often, when we thought we were lost. It is a time when we may discover or remember once again that this human journey is much easier when we love one another, see the divinity in each other, and know we are not alone.

I have often ended a lecture or workshop by playing a simple song called "All This Joy" by John Denver, because his words tell it all—they tell us about the ingredients of life and the fullness of it. I suggest you read it slowly, out loud to yourself.

> *All this joy, all this sorrow, all this promise, all this pain.*
> *Such is life, such is being, such is spirit, such is love.*[4]

Love to you.

---

4. John Denver, "All This Joy," from the album *Higher Ground* (Windstar Records, 1990).

ACKNOWLEDGMENTS

The publication date for *Close to the Bone* is October 2, 1996. I think of this day as a special day, a day that acknowledges and celebrates the entry of a new book that will go out into the world and have a life of its own. I think about an equivalent celebration that announced and welcomed a newborn child in ancient Greece. It also took place after the actual birth. On this day, the infant was carried three times around Hestia's sacred fire. As Goddess of the Hearth and Temple, her essence was in the fire at the center of a round hearth; an image that came to mind when I saw the Scribner symbol on the first page of this book, flames in a round hearth.

I have been warmly welcomed into the family of Scribner authors. My thanks to Leigh Haber, my editor, whose suggestions were valuable and whose enthusiasm was contagious, and to her assistant, Kristina Nwazota; to John Fontana, who designed the beautiful cover; to Jennifer Dossin and Margery Cantor for the interior design of the book; to Susan Moldow, my publisher, who supported this book from the beginning and went to bat for the Georgia O'Keeffe painting on the cover; and to Pat Eisemann, Roz Lippel, and Sharon Dynak for their part.

My thanks to Jan Adrian, whose visionary work began and sustained the "Healing Journeys: Cancer as a Turning Point" conferences, with the help of Anna Kreck, Merrily Bronson, and Mickey Angello. Her invitations to speak about cancer as a soul experience to hundreds of women with cancer led me to writing *Close to the Bone*. Others contributed to this book in many different ways. I thank Patricia Ellerd Demetrios, Ann Chappell, Jan Lovett-Keen, Beth Milwid, Mollie Schardt, Michael Steele, Anthea Francine, my father, Joseph Shinoda, my mother, Megumi Y. Shinoda, my son, Andre Bolen, Dwight McKee, Betty Grayson, Betty Karr, and many unnamed individuals who shared their stories with me.

I was delighted when I heard that October 2 is the Guardian Angel day on the Catholic calendar. It felt like a blessing, as synchronicities do, and only a person whose birthday it was could have known and told me. Since I think that when we pray for others, an angel goes to sit on their shoulders, then maybe a guardian angel will come to you with this book. For this book is like a prayer, meant to help and heal, to make you less afraid, to encourage you to trust the wisdom that is inside. It is a soul-to-soul communication, and guardian angels may very well accompany intentions such as these.

SOURCES

Frankl, Viktor E. *Man's Search for Meaning: An Introduction to Logotherapy.* Translated by Ilse Lasch. New York: Pocket Books, 1963.

Hirshberg, Caryle, and Marc Ian Barasch. *Remarkable Recovery: What Extraordinary Healings Tell Us About Getting Well and Staying Well.* New York: Riverhead Books, 1995.

Lerner, Michael. *Choices in Healing: Integrating the Best of Conventional and Complementary Approaches to Cancer.* Cambridge, Mass.: MIT Press, 1994.

LeShan, Lawrence. *Cancer as a Turning Point: A Handbook for People with Cancer, Their Families, and Health Professionals.* Revised edition. New York: Plume, Penguin Books USA, 1994.

Ornish, Dean. *Dr. Dean Ornish's Program for Reversing Heart Disease: The Only System Scientifically Proven to Reverse Heart Disease Without Drugs or Surgery.* New York: Ballantine, 1990.

Siegel, Bernie S. *Love, Medicine and Miracles: Lessons Learned About Self-Healing from a Surgeon's Experience with Exceptional Patients.* New York: Harper & Row, 1986.

Simonton, O. Carl, Stephanie Matthews-Simonton, and James L. Creighton. *Getting Well Again: A Step-by-Step, Self-Help Guide to Overcoming Cancer for Patients and Their Families.* New York: Bantam, 1980.

Weil, Andrew. *Spontaneous Healing: How to Discover and Enhance Your Body's Natural Ability to Maintain and Heal Itself.* New York: Knopf, 1995.

INDEX

abandonment:
    and dismemberment, 64, 65–66
    fear of, 116
    of patient, 50, 116
abusive relationships, 53–54, 192
Achterberg, Jeanne, 138
addictions:
    as escape, 18, 55, 71
    illness as escape from, 72
Adrian, Jan, 155–56
affirmations, 152–56
    in recovery, 143–44
    three Vs in, 156
AIDS:
    and healing stories, 106–8
    and holding the opposites, 201
    hospices for, 73–75
    and Inanna-Ereshkigal myth, 58–60
    and loving sacrifice, 120
    response to, 35–36
    and shadow of death, 36–38
    and support groups, 125
    and survival, 107
    and warrior marks, 49–50
alchemy:
    of prayer, 142
    of sculpture, 83
Alcoholics Anonymous, 139, 193–94

allergies, ridding body of, 104–5
allopathic medicine:
    aggressive methods of, 102–3
    experimental protocol in, 106
    as "guy thing," 143
    and turning point, 85
"All This Joy" (Denver), 210
alternative therapies:
    ignorance of, 100–101
    and self-healing, 102–3
    stories of, 106
anecdotal evidence, 100
angels:
    and prayer, 130, 141
    visits of, 13–14
    white cells as, 148–49
Angels in America (Kushner), 118–19
Anthea:
    and Inanna myth, 173–75
    and post-surgery rituals, 168–70
    and ritual in operating room, 166–67
Appointment in Samarra (O'Hara), 203–4
archetypes, 78–79
    Ereshkigal, 56
    and journey, 180
    meaning of sacrifice in, 177
    of meaning within us, 142
    of midwife, 207

archetypes (*cont.*)
    in stories, 109
Athens, as symbolic destination, 63–64

Bannister, Roger, 104, 105
Barasch, Marc Ian, 122, 190
belief:
    archetypal, 113–15
    and healing, 105
    in magic, 97
    and prayer, 130–33, 139
    in recovery, 99–100, 128
    in stories, 92, 97, 98, 103, 105–6, 109,
        144–45
    and suffering, 94
    in survival, 196–97
    testing of, 206
Beyond Love (Lapierre), 140–41
biting the bullet, 40
bliss and harmony, 77–79
Bly, Robert, 189
bodhisattva, 191
body:
    communication of soul and, 106
    healing system of, 94–95, 98, 100–101,
        102–3
Bohm, David, 152
brain, and repetition, 152–53
Brenman-Gibson, Margaret, 191
Bridge of San Luis Rey, The (Wilder), 203
Brown, Daniel, 191, 192
Brown, Jerry, 74
Buber, Martin, 115
Byrd, Richard, 131

Campbell, Joseph, 51, 77–78
cancer:
    and abandonment, 50
    and archetypal meaning of sacrifice, 177
    as death wish, 169
    and LeShan, 76–77, 80, 81–83
    and loving sacrifice, 120
    and macrobiotics, 99–100
    and meditation, 145–46
    and mind-body connection, 102–3, 145–46
    "Mr. Wright" and dissolving tumor, 95–98
    and psychological impact of diagnosis, 84
    and psychotherapy, 145
    remission of, 85, 97–98, 103
    and shadow of death, 36–38
    support groups, 125
    and Therapeutic Touch, 134
    as turning point, 76–77, 155–56, 190
    and visualization, 103, 145–47
    as wake-up call, 41, 51–52
    and warrior marks, 49–50

Cancer as a Turning Point (LeShan), 76–77
cells:
    communication from mind to, 108–9
        and DNA, 109
    receptors in, 94–95
    and visualization, 147
chemotherapy:
    effects of, 100
    and physical appearance, 37
    as ritual, 170–72
    and underworld, 45
    and warrior marks, 49–50
Choices in Healing (Lerner), 135
Christianity, and Eleusinian Mysteries, 208–9
Christmas Carol, A (Dickens), 188
Commonweal Cancer Help Program, 74–75,
    135–36
compassion:
    and action, 191–93
    and Dalai Lama, 191–92
    and gratitude, 182
    and grief, 189–90
    as healing force, 187
    and helping others, 179–80, 192–93
    illness and, 210
    vs. indifference, 192
    and self-healing, 190–91
    and suffering, 184–85, 186–87, 189
    as turning point, 180
concentration camps, 34–35, 37–38
connection, see I-Thou relationships
consciousness, matter preceded by, 95
control:
    circumstances beyond, 195–96
    ego and, 34
    loss of, 22
Cousins, Norman, 183–84
creativity:
    and collective unconscious, 26
    foiled, 80
    inner sources of, 80–81, 82
    and *kairos*, 86–88
    search for, 83
    and work, 88
    see also imagination
crone figures, 208
Crossing to Avalon (Bolen), 109, 133
Crow and Weasel (Lopez), 109
crucible, relationships in, 118–20

Dalai Lama, 191–92
dance, prayer expressed through, 133–34
death:
    and dreams, 20
    and ego, 209
    fear of, 62

living in shadow of, 36–38
as metaphor, 33
mystery of, 15
readiness for, 205
and resurrection, 33, 164
symbolic, 55
time and place for, 203–5
as transition, 169, 209
wishes for, 68, 169
de Decker, Jacqueline, 140–41
defenses, dissolution of, 31
Demeter, and Persephone, 126–28, 181–82, 193, 207, 208
denial:
of Ereshkigal qualities, 62
of suffering, 179
unconscious operation of, 122
and underworld, 32
depression:
end of, 182
and immune system, 43, 50, 102
and loss of psychological defenses, 31
and repression, 56, 58, 67
suicidal, 112
underworld of, 25–26, 53, 56
Dickens, Charles, 188
diet, macrobiotic, 99–100, 102–3
Dionysus, 165
disease, *see* illness
dismemberment:
and Procrustes, 63
and recovery, 65–66
divinity, experience of, 132
doctors:
communication from, 38–39
defensive medicine of, 92
like generals at war, 15
optimism of, 98, 101, 156
and patient relationship, 68, 92–94
and positive emotional response, 94–95
Dossey, Larry, 131, 132
Dr. Dean Ornish's Program for Reversing Heart Disease (Ornish), 85*n*
dreams:
aborted, 80–81
and collective unconscious, 26
of continuity, 209
insights from, 210
interpretation of, 26–27
and soul realm, 19, 20, 26
Dumbo and his magic feather, 97

earthquakes, real and metaphorical, 201–2
East West Foundation, 99
ego:
and control, 34

and death, 209
descent of, 62
in outer-directed life, 70
in prayer, 142
and procrustean bed, 65
and underworld, 81
Eleusinian Mysteries, 208–9
Eliot, T. S., 114, 181, 209
emotions, *see* feelings
energy:
healing, 136–38
spiritual, 19
transmission of, 138, 144
and visualization, 146
Engler, Jack, 191
Ereshkigal:
as archetype, 56
identification with, 61–62
as Inanna's sister, 29, 54
integrating strengths of, 66–67
and release from pain, 60
suffering of, 29, 54, 56, 57, 58, 62, 64, 186
transformation of, 66, 185–86
underworld of, 29, 32–33, 34
Erickson, Erik, 181
ESP, 147
evil, and Hades, 24
expectations:
and emotion-colored pictures, 156
and healing, 91, 94
and hexes, 91
and illness, 88, 91
and *kronos*, 87–88
procrustean bed of, 63–64, 65
prognoses as, 196
reality vs., 122
unfulfilled, 198

faith, ordeal of, 206
Fantasia (Disney), 150
fear:
of abandonment, 116
absence of, 172
of cancer, 84
of engulfment, 123
and Ereshkigal myth, 62
illness and, 17, 94
of loss, 116
and love, 121
of rejection, 62
repression of, 26
underworld of, 24–25
feelings:
and dismemberment, 64
and Ereshkigal myth, 66
expression of, 67

feelings (*cont.*)
    hidden, 26, 117
    repression of, 26, 56–58, 67, 189
    in soul moments, 17–18
"Fellowship of Those Who Bear the Mark of
    Pain, The" (Schweitzer), 182, 184, 186,
    192, 208
Four Quartets (Eliot), 114, 181, 209
Frankl, Viktor, 34–35, 37, 116

Getting Well Again (Simonton), 144–47
Getty, Jeff, 106–7
Gift of the Sea (Lindbergh), 47
gnosis, 43–44
Goddesses in Everywoman (Bolen), 78, 206
Gods in Everyman (Bolen), 78
Goleman, Daniel, 191
grace, defined, 73
gratitude:
    and compassion, 182
    for gift of life, 69, 180
    for loyal friendship, 163–64
    for sacrifice, 120
grief:
    and compassion, 189–90
    contaminated experience of, 200
    for loss of health, 206
"Guardian Angel Prayer, The," 139–40
Guo Ling, 190

Hades:
    and evil, 24
    and Persephone, 23–24, 91, 126, 181-82
    and underworld, 23–24, 26, 44
hands, laying on of, 49
hands-on healing, 134–38
harmony and bliss, 77–79
Hay, Louise L., 153–54, 205–6
Head, Phil, 37
healing:
    and bedside manner, 92–95
    and belief, 104
    and expectations, 91, 95
    hands-on, 49, 134–38
    and immune system, 76
    as inner shift, 187
    integrated experience of, 207
    and love, 82–83, 134–35
    miraculous, 98
    mourning in, 206
    nature's power of, 93
    neutrality vs., 93–94
    and prayer, 71, 129–42
    and psychotherapy, 82–83
    ritual of, 157–60
    self-, *see* self-healing

    of the soul, 71
    from stories, 95–98, 106–7, 108, 143–44
    as subjective response, 170
    by touch, 134–35
    see also recovery
healing circles, 71–73, 123–25
    hospices, 73–74, 75
    information shared in, 124–25
    I-Thou relationships in, 73, 123–25
    and remission, 85
    sanctuary of, 123–25, 159
    unconditional love in, 73–75
Healing Journeys, 155
Healing Words (Dossey), 131, 132
heart:
    dissolving shell around, 188–91
    sacrifice from, 119–20
    and underworld's riches, 81–82
heart attacks, as wake-up calls, 41
heart disease:
    reversal of, 85, 151
    and visualization, 151–52
Hecate, 207–8
Hermes (Mercury), 13, 91–92, 105–9, 182
heroes, and warrior marks, 49–50
Hestia, Goddess of Hearth and Temple, 72
hexes, and expectations, 91
Hirshberg, Caryle, 122, 190
hope:
    of recovery, 94, 96–98
    of resurrection, 55
Hopkins, Pat, 129
Hospice for the Destitute and Dying, 73–74
hospital:
    and concentration camp, 37
    and discriminating actions, 47–49
    entry into underworld and, 30–31, 38–39
    line of authority in, 14
    preparation for, 163
    ritual in, 166–67, 175
    as village, 184–85
    and visitors, 47–49
hot coals, walking barefoot on, 104, 105
humiliation, from disease and treatment, 94
humor, 37–38

illness:
    as close to the bone, 21–22
    and compassion, 210
    as descent into underworld, 23–39, 61–62
    and detente, 84–86
    diagnosis of, 16
    as enemy, 15, 143
    as escape, 68
    and expectations, 88, 94
    as initiation, 157

and innocence, 74
invasive treatments for, 16
isolation and, 125, 136
as life-altering passage, 182–84
liminal time and place, 15–16
line from health to, 14
and loss of control, 22
as mind- and life-threatening, 70
and moments of truth, 116–17
progression of, 85, 206
as psychological ordeal, 17
questions raised by, 70
recurrence of, 111, 113
remission of, 85, 97, 100, 103
resistance to, 136
and the soul, 14–15, 19, 21, 41–42, 70–71, 210
as spiritual journey, 115–16, 178
as test, 115, 205–6
as time out, 89
tipping the scales of, 131–32
and transformation, 19, 65, 67
turning point of, 28, 67, 69, 76–90, 180
as wake-up call, 40–41, 45–52
and "why me?," 197–99
see also specific diseases
imagination, 143–56
in affirmations, 156
and healing stories, 143–44
and immune system, 147–49
power of, 95
see also creativity; visualization
immune system:
and chemotherapy, 100
and depression, 43, 50, 102
and healing, 76
and macrobiotics, 103
and mind-body connection, 146
and prayer, 140
and visualization, 102–3, 147–49
Inanna, 29–32, 53–62
and approval, 57
Ereshkigal as sister of, 29, 54
identification with, 54, 56, 57, 61–62
Ninshubur as loyal friend of, 58–59, 66, 126, 127, 163
and psychotherapy, 55
resurrection of, 60, 66–67, 126
and suffering, 33–34, 53, 61–62
individuation:
and archetypal journey, 180
and personal truth, 82
and procrustean bed, 65
information:
and psyche, 109
sharing of, 124–25

in stories, 105, 107
initiation:
blood mystery, 157
Inanna myth and, 60
and transformation of suffering, 33
inner wisdom (gnosis), 43–44, 152
Institute of Noetics Sciences, 98
Iron John (Bly), 189
isolation, 125, 136
I-Thou relationships:
coining expression of, 113
doctor and patient, 92–94
and hands-on healing, 135
as lifelines, 112–13, 123, 125
motherhood, 133–34
mutuality in, 120–21
and prayer, 140–41
risks in, 122
in ritual, 158
of soul companions, 110, 112–13, 121, 140

Jesus, and transformation of suffering, 33–34
Job, 197
journey:
archetypal, 180
medical, 33–34, 51
in mythology, 51, 52
spiritual, 33, 62, 88, 115–16
Jung, C. G., 78, 109, 115

kairos, 86–87, 88
Klopfer, Bruno, 95–96
Krieger, Dolores, 135
kronos, 86, 87–88
Kushner, Tony, 118–19

Lapierre, Dominique, 140–41
Lerner, Michael, 135–36
LeShan, Lawrence, 76–77
and creativity, 80
positive focus of, 81–83
and turning point, 84–85, 190
Levine, Stephen, 185–86, 188,
life:
affirmation of, 169
applying mythology to, 47
creative, 81
enhancement and extension of, 76, 83, 125
gift of, 69, 180
illness as alteration of, 182–84
meaningful, 81, 181
outer-directed, 70
purpose of, 82
and self-discovery, 77
as short and precious, 15, 16, 181, 210
of significant soil, 180–81

life (*cont.*)
    as soul journey, 88
    span of, 204
    spiritual perspective of, 114
    tests of, 206
    and turning point, 85
    as unpredictable, 196
    and wake-up call, 50–51
    wild and precious, 89, 181
    work as center of, 72
liminal experience, 15–16
Lindbergh, Anne Morrow, 47
Link for the Sick and Suffering Coworkers of
        Mother Teresa, 141, 142
Little Engine That Could, The, 143–44, 152
Lopez, Barry, 109
love:
    as expressed in prayer, 142
    and fear, 121
    and healing, 82–83, 134–35
    and I-Thou relationships, 115, 120–21
    and lifelines, 113
    and risk, 121
    and sacrifice, 120
    and self-healing, 154
    and survival, 127
    and time, 86
    and turning point, 180
    unconditional, 73–75
Love, Medicine and Miracles (Siegel), 67–68

macrobiotics, 99–100, 102–3
Macy, Joanna, 191
magic:
    belief in, 97
    of ritual words, 172–76
Man's Search for Meaning (Frankl), 34–35
matter, preceded by consciousness, 95, 105
meditation:
    and cancer, 145–46
    clearing one's mind for, 87
    and inner nature, 71
    and openness, 27, 178
    and reversal of disease, 85
    and ritual, 178
    and visualization, 148–49, 150
memories:
    forgotten, 76
    and healing, 65
    of pleasures, 79
    and psychotherapy, 71
    of recurring illness, 111
    as sources of meaning, 88
    and underworld, 32
Mercury (Hermes), 13, 91–92, 105–8, 182
metaphors:

Athens, 63–64
    death, 33
    earthquakes, 201–4
    East, 55
    illness as descent into underworld, 24, 61–62
    journey, 51, 52, 88, 162–64
    lamp and knife, 42–43, 52
    pomegranate seeds, 193
    procrustean bed, 63
    stories as, 105
    uses of, 24, 43–44, 177
    visualization of, 144–45
Michelangelo, 83
midwife:
    archetype of, 207
    to the soul, 134–35
mind-body connection, 105, 109, 170
    and affirmations, 152
    and alternative therapies, 102–3
    and stories, 98
    and visualization, 145–46, 147
Missionaries of Charity, 140–41
morphic field, 109, 138, 139–40
Mother Earth, 133
mountain climbing, and survival, 125
multiple personalities, 104–5
music:
    deeply heard, 86
    prayer expressed through, 133–34
    in ritual, 175, 176
mutuality, 120–21; *see also* I-Thou relationships
mythology:
    and Eleusinian Mysteries, 208–9
    Ereshkigal, 29, 32–33, 34, 56
    finding your own, 77–78
    Hades (Pluto), 23–24, 26, 44
    Hermes (Mercury), 91–92, 105–9
    Inanna, 29–32, 33–34, 53–62
    Jesus, 33–34
    Ninshubur, 58–59
    Persephone, 23–24, 29, 91, 181–82
    and perspective, 38
    Psyche, 41–43, 44, 51, 52
    and rituals, 157–78
    and truth, 78
    uses of, 43–44, 46–47, 60, 128, 210
    Zeus, 165, 182

"Namaste," 121, 172
natural disasters, 196, 201–4
nature, healing power of, 93
near death experiences, 28–29
"Neuropeptides and Their Receptors" (Pert),
        94–95
neutrality vs. healing, 93–94
Niebuhr, Reinhold, 139

Ninshubur, and Inanna, 58–59, 66, 126, 127, 163
"No!":
    and discriminating actions, 47–49
    and moments of truth, 45
    and personal meaning, 45–47
    and Psyche myth, 44–45, 47
Nussbaum, Elaine, 99–101, 190–91

O'Hara, John, 203–4
Oliver, Mary, 89
Ornish, Dean, 85, 151

pain:
    and biting the bullet, 40
    and compassion, 187
    as connection to others, 187
    from disease and treatment, 94
    and Ereshkigal, 58, 60, 62, 66
    repression of, 56–57, 189
    self-hypnosis for, 124
    transformation of, 33
    withdrawal from, 55, 64
    witnesses to, 60
parapsychology, 147
patient:
    abandonment of, 50, 116
    activist, 68, 107
    anonymity of, 92
    and bedside visits, 47–49
    blame placed on, 50, 197, 199–200
    death wishes of, 68
    and doctor relationship, 68, 92–94
    exceptional, 67–68, 147, 199
    good, 14–15, 16, 25, 26
    and Inanna myth, 30–31
    infantilizing of, 25
    lawsuit from, 92
    mental change in, 154
    physical appearance of, 37
    positive focus on, 81–83
    powerlessness of, 94
    and Psyche myth, 51
    rage of, 198–99
    "red blanket," 38
    risks for, 115–16, 117
    self-healing abilities of, *see* self-healing
    shameful feelings of, 111
    stories of and for, 95–98
    uniqueness of, 82
Patricia:
    and elements of remission, 101-3
    and hair-cutting ritual, 158-60
    and chemo-therapy ritual, 170-71
peptides, 94–95, 102–3
Persephone, 23–24, 29, 91, 105–6

    and Demeter, 126–28, 181–82, 193, 207, 208
    and Hades, 23–24, 91, 126, 181
    and Hecate, 207–8
Pert, Candace, 94–95
Pluto, Lord of the Underworld, 26
Power Is Within You, The (Hay), 153
prana energy, 135, 138
prayer, 129–42
    alchemy of, 142
    and angels, 129–30, 142
    and belief, 130–31, 139
    and centeredness, 130
    to divine mystery and source, 129–30, 132–33
    ego in, 142
    and healing, 71, 129–42
    healing touch as, 134–35
    and immune system, 140
    and I-Thou links, 140–41
    love expressed in, 142
    and meaning of life, 209–10
    physical expressions of, 133–34
    receptiveness in, 26
    repeated, 138–40
    and ritual, 178
    soul links of, 140–41
    for survival, 129
Price, Reynolds, 150, 197–98
priorities:
    close-to-the-bone concerns, 21
    shifting of, 15–16, 34, 70, 123–24, 180
procrustean bed, 63–65
Procrustes, 63
psyche:
    communication from, 27
    and death, 209
    and denial, 40
    and information, 109
    living contents of, 65
    and recovery, 100
    and ritual, 172
    and visualization, 151–52
Psyche:
    journey of, 52
    myth of, 41–43, 44, 51
    personal meaning of, 45–47
    and saying "No!," 44–45, 47, 49
psychotherapy:
    alchemy of, 83
    and cancer, 145
    and healing, 82–83
    and Inanna myth, 55
    as lifeline, 112
    negative focus of, 81
    and remembering, 71

qi energy, 135, 138

radiation therapy:
  and physical appearance, 37
  ritual of, 165
  and underworld, 44–45
  and visualization, 146
  and warrior marks, 50
rebirth, *see* resurrection
recovery:
  affirmations in, 143
  belief in, 99, 100, 128
  of dismembered parts, 65–66
  and expectations, 91
  as gift of life, 68, 180
  and giving back to society, 180, 190
  hope of, 94, 96–98
  of innocence, 74
  from I-Thou relationships, 123
  miraculous, 98, 100
  myths of, 126–28
  positive emotional response and, 94–95, 144
  from powerful inward experiences, 122
  and repression, 69
  ritual of, 164
  and Serenity Prayer, 139
  support groups, 193–94
  visualization in, 143, 145
  see also healing
Recovery: From Cancer to Health through Macro-
  biotics (Nussbaum), 99, 190–91
reincarnation, of bodhisattva, 191
rejection:
  and dismemberment, 64
  fear of, 62
  tumor as symbol of, 168
relationships:
  abusive, 53–54, 192
  in crucible, 118–20
  divine, 129–30
  I-Thou, *see* I-Thou relationships
  and loving sacrifice, 120
  mutuality in, 120–21
  procrustean bed of, 63
  soul-consuming, 70–71, 72
remembering, *see* memories
remission:
  and belief in stories, 103
  miraculous, 100–101
  possibility of, 85, 97
repression:
  and Ereshkigal myth, 66
  of feelings, 26, 56–58, 67, 189
  and recovery, 69
response:
  and character, 36, 52
  choice of, 35–36, 116, 117
  positive emotional, 94–95, 144

  subjective, 170
resurrection:
  death and, 33, 164
  and the East, 55
  hope of, 55
  of Inanna, 60, 66–67, 126
  of personal meaning and truth, 82–83
  symbolic, 55, 62, 168
  transformation of, 209
  tree planting as symbol of, 168
reverie, *see* dreams
Rhine, J. B., 147
rituals, 157–78
  blood mysteries, 157
  chemotherapy as, 170–72
  created vs. traditional, 158
  elements of, 161–62
  everyday, 176
  of healing, 158–60
  of hospital entry, 157–58
  instinct for, 158–60
  and letting go of the past, 176
  magic of words in, 172–76
  and meditation, 178
  and metaphor of journey, 162–64
  in operating room, 166–67
  post-surgery, 168–70
  and prayer, 178
  prior to surgery, 160
  rites of passage, 52
  sacrifice or scapegoat in, 176–78
  and sanctuary space, 171–72
  and soul, 178
  telling of the story in, 161
  transformation in, 33, 159, 164, 168
  tree planting as rebirth, 168

sacrifice:
  archetypal meaning of, 177
  from the heart, 119–20
  and love, 120
  in rituals, 176–78
St. Andrews, Barbara, 203
sanctuary:
  of healing circles, 71–72, 123–25, 159
  of I-Thou relationships, 121–22
  in ritual, 171–72
Sattilaro, Anthony, 99
Schweitzer, Albert, 182–83, 184, 185, 186, 192, 208
Scrooge, Ebenezer, 188
self-esteem:
  low, 56, 88
  and productivity, 79
self-healing:
  and alternative therapies, 102–3
  and bedside manner, 93

body's system for, 94–95, 98, 100, 102–3
and compassion, 190–91
focus on, 81–82, 97
and love, 154
and visualization, 150
Serenity Prayer, 139
Sheldrake, Rupert, 109
Siegel, Bernie, 67–68
Simonton, O. Carl, 102, 145–47, 148, 150
Smith, Helene, 60–61
soul:
    alchemy of, 83
    and angel's visit, 13–15
    asking questions of, 169
    and authenticity, 69
    baring of, 18
    bodhisattva, 191
    comfort for, 74
    communication of body and, 106
    connections of, *see* soul connections
    dissolving shell around, 188–91
    and grace, 73
    growth of, 41–42
    healing of, 71
    home from a journey, 205
    and illness, 14–15, 19, 21, 41–42, 70–71, 210
    journey of, 33, 62, 88
    language of, 24, 33, 43
    midwife to, 134–35
    questions of, 19–20
    reaction to loss by, 206
    realm of, 14, 19
    replenishment of, 142
    revelation of, 178
    underworld of, 26–27, 81
soul connections, 110–28
    and archetypal beliefs, 113–15
    and circles of support, 123–25
    crucible of, 118–20
    I-Thou, 110, 112–13, 121–23, 140
    and moments of truth, 116–17
    mutuality of, 120–21
    and recovery myths, 126–28
    and recurring illness, 111
    and spiritual journey, 115–16
soul level, 18–19, 115
    choices, 34–35
    turning point, 85
Spiegel, David, 123–25
Spontaneous Remission (Institute of Noetics Sciences), 98
Starhawk, 174
stories, 91–109
    belief in, 92, 97–99, 103, 105, 106, 109, 144
    case histories as, 98–99

healing power of, 95–98, 106–7, 108, 143–44
identification with, 95, 99–101
information in, 105, 107
insights from, 46
inspirational, 144
as metaphors, 105
of miraculous recovery, 98–99, 100
and ritual, 161
sources of, 95
visualization of, 144–45
see also mythology
Stress, Diet and Your Heart (Ornish), 151
stress reduction, 151
suffering:
    compassion in midst of, 184–85, 187, 189
    as cross to bear, 113–14
    denial of, 179
    with disease and treatment, 94
    of Ereshkigal, 29, 54, 56, 57, 58, 62, 66, 186
    and Inanna myth, 33–34, 54, 61–62
    integration of, 193
    meaningless, 94
    offering of, 141, 142
    perspective on, 38, 94
    redemption of, 193
    transformation of, 33–35, 142, 186–87
    universality of, 179, 198
support groups, 124–25
    and heart disease, 151–52
    and recovery, 193–94
    and remission, 85
    and ritual, 161
    see also healing circles
surgery:
    and archetypal meaning of sacrifice, 177
    and biting the bullet, 40
    parallels to initiation, 164–65
    and post-surgery rituals, 168–71
    and ritual in operating room, 166–67
    rituals prior to, 160
survival:
    AIDS and, 107
    belief in, 196–97
    and doctor-patient relationship, 68
    and healing circles, 124
    to keep on keeping on, 110, 113, 125, 206
    and love, 127
    prayer for, 129
    purpose of, 180
    vs. thriving, 41

talents:
    innate, 79–80
    repression of, 57

talents (*cont.*)
    uncultivated, 81
    and work, 88
temenos (sanctuary), 71
    of healing circles, 123–25, 159
    of I-Thou relationship, 121–22
Teresa, Mother, 73, 140–41, 142
Therapeutic Touch, 135–36
time, 86–88
transformation:
    of Ereshkigal, 66, 185–86
    illness and, 19, 65, 67
    of resurrection, 209
    in ritual, 33, 159, 164, 168
    in soul realm, 19
    of suffering, 33–34, 142, 185–86
    transpersonal element in, 185
truth:
    and bliss, 78–79
    finding your own, 80–82
    and I-Thou relationships, 122
    moments of, 45, 116–17
    and myth, 77
    resurrection of, 82–83
    at soul level, 19
Truth or Dare (Starhawk), 174
turning point, 28, 34, 67, 69
    and achieving detente, 84–86
    and alternative therapies, 85
    archetypes in, 78–79
    cancer as, 76–77, 155–56, 190
    compassion as, 180
    and finding your myth, 77–78
    and finding your path, 89–90
    and finding your truth, 82–83
    and inner sources of creative life, 80
    and search for meaning, 85–86, 88
Twenty-third Psalm, 169–70

unconscious:
    collective, 26, 81, 109, 138, 169
    and denial, 122
    dismembered parts in, 66
    inner world of, 70
    and underworld, 26–27
underworld:
    and denial, 32
    of depression, 24–26, 53, 56
    entry into, 30–31, 38–39, 157–58
    Hades as Lord of, 23–24, 26
    Hermes as messenger of, 13, 91–92
    illness as descent into, 23–39, 61–62
    Inanna's descent into, 29–32, 54–55
    and memory, 32
    Pluto as Lord of, 24

Psyche's descent into, 44
    return from, 193–94, 207
    of shadow and depth, 32–33
    of the soul, 26–27
    of the spirits, 28–29
    and treatments, 44–45

visualization, 144–52
    and allergy, 105
    and arthritis, 147
    and cancer, 102, 145–47
    emotion-colored pictures in, 156
    and heart disease, 151–52
    images in, 148, 151
    and immune system, 102–3, 147–49
    and meditation, 148, 150
    and physiological changes, 149–50
    in recovery, 143, 145–46
    and self-healing, 150
vulnerability:
    and baring the soul, 18
    illness and, 17, 25, 71
    and I-Thou relationships, 120–21, 122
    and prayer, 129

Walker, Alice, 52, 133
Walsh, Gary, 28–29
warrior marks, 49–50
Welwood, John, 152
"We Shall Overcome," 175
When the Worst That Can Happen Already Has
    (Head), 37
Whole New Life, A (Price), 198
"why me?," 197–99
wisdom (gnosis), 43–44
    cellular, 94
    philosophical restatements of, 113
wish to die, 68, 169
wish to live, 50–51
women:
    approval sought by, 57, 58
    feelings repressed by, 56
Woodman, Marion, 137–38
work:
    addiction to, 72
    and creativity, 88
    and *kronos*, 87–88
    procrustean bed of, 63
worthlessness, sense of, 56, 58
"Wright, Mr.," 95–98

yoga, and reversal of disease, 85
You Can Heal Your Life (Hay), 153

Zeus, 126, 165, 181